Sweet

Nectar

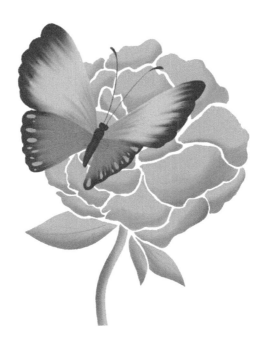

Sweet Nectar:

(Hopefully) *Everything You Want To Know About Chestfeeding*

Kylia P. Kennedy

Certified Breastfeeding Specialist, Lactation Education Resources
Cover Illustration by Safiya Yasmeen

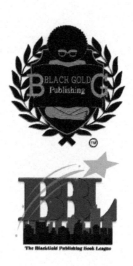

**Published by BlackGold Publishing, LLC in partnership with
The BlackGold Book League of Hampton Roads.**

1706 Todds Lane, Suite 258
Hampton, VA 23666

Edited by: Johnnae Roberts
Formatted by: J. Matthews
Copyright © 2021 by Kylia P. Kennedy
First Edition: April 2022
Printed in the United States of America

"Late at night when the room was dark and cool and the world around us was silent, all the troubles of the day melted away..."

"This was home, not a place but a feeling..."

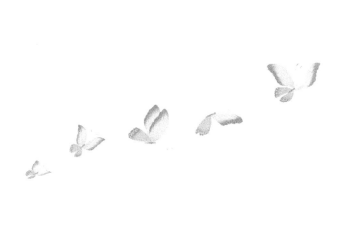

Dedication &
Acknowledgements

This book is dedicated to my *sweet petit papillon* and my incredible husband, both for their unwavering and unconditional patience, love and support throughout this entire process. To my mother for always reminding me that I can do anything with a lot of work, creativity, patience, and perseverance. To my best friends, Aubrey and Sean, for giving me space to take up space and for never letting me forget how much I deserve to have my story told. To my best friend, Marianne, for constantly telling me how proud they are of me, giving me so many words of affirmation and for creating the subtitle for this book. And lastly, to all of my twitter followers, for being an ever encouraging presence throughout my entire journey. When I didn't know if Aubrey would ever latch again, when I was searching for parents to include in this book, when I needed help deciding what to include in part three, when I felt overwhelmed with the road ahead-- they never failed to support and encourage me. This community of "strangers" became a family to me and I truly could not and would not have pushed as long and as hard as I did if not for them.

I am eternally grateful.

Table of Contents

Table of Contents
(continued)

Foreword

This is a story I started writing before I knew how it would end. Yes, we all love a good "happy ending," but life doesn't always work out that way and that's okay. Regardless of how this story ends, I'm just happy to be telling it. This book goes into the many challenges I faced as a young, breastfeeding mother in an ill-informed society that pushed formula on me every chance it got.

When this all started, my daughter didn't need formula, she needed her mother to be supported by informed doctors, family and friends. I know there are parents out there who may very well be going through the same thing, or maybe already did and felt alone or voiceless. It was very important to me to separate this book into three parts. The first part being my story, told from my point of view-- raw and real. The second, a compilation of stories, just the same. The third, an educational section, where I give valuable information that will help you advocate for yourself and others. This book is inclusive, nursing knows no gender, no age, no race or religion. I hope that this is reflected in part III. Though the terms "breastfeeding" and "mother" resonate with me and many of the parents in part II, I have written part III with inclusive and approachable language.

To you, reading this, *you are not alone and I will be your voice*. I believe your story. I believe how the doctors treated you. I believe the emotions you felt. I believe the nights you spent crying and wondering why you weren't enough. I believe you. I hear you. We are one.

Kylia Kennedy,
United States, They/She

Sweet Nectar Part I – *My Story*

Prologue - Circa 2000-2018

Long before I ever thought about having children, I knew I wanted to breastfeed. I had seen my mother do it for my three younger siblings, so I had plenty of exposure to it. I remember my mother making it look so easy and effortless. She frequently told me the story of how when I was about four-years-old I would put my baby dolls to my nipple and pretend to nurse them. In high school I remember looking up, "How to Breastfeed" on Google and in college I was always so amazed and inspired when I saw a woman nursing in public. It amazed me how powerful breast milk is and I couldn't wait to say that I had nursed my (future) children well after infancy.

When my husband and I finally got pregnant, I asked the few moms I knew what I should add to our baby registry. I often got suggestions like "bottles," "bottle warmer," "formula," and always overlooked those because I never even wanted to have to pump for our daughter.

At our baby shower, we received a handmade lamp from one of my husband's stepsisters. When I opened it, I was thrilled and said "Oh this will be perfect for those late night nursing sessions!" One of our guests responded with "Oh, you're going to breastfeed?" I answered with, "Of course." There was never a moment of doubt in my mind; I wanted to nurse all of our children, I was determined to. Never in a million years did I think I would struggle through nursing the first one. Not a single family member or friend, Facebook group or birthing class prepared me for my personal version of hell. How could they have? I learned over the course of less than a year that the vast majority of "experienced parents," nurses and doctors haven't the slightest idea of how lactation actually works. So, when we ran into obstacles, I set out for my own answers… *and now I'm sharing them with you.*

April 2019

At 4:40 am on Friday, April 12, 2019, my husband and I were wide awake, packing the car for a day that felt like it would never come: my induction day. We did one last check around the house to make sure we hadn't forgotten any essentials... my bathrobe, our toothbrushes, the stroller... We said goodbye to our fur babies and set off for the hospital.

As we made our way through the Emergency Room to the Labor and Delivery wing, I felt the butterflies start to really take flight. Adrenaline, anxiety, and anticipation all played a role that day. The culmination of nine months of daydreaming about what our daughter would look like, painting the nursery, stocking up on tiny socks and doing research on how to have the picture perfect breastfeeding journey was finally mere hours away from us. We took some time to settle into our room, sign paperwork and meet the day shift staff.

When 8:00 am rolled around, the Pitocin started dripping. At that moment, I felt ready. I began to practice accepting the great surges of energy as one step closer to holding my baby in my arms. It wasn't long before the surges really started building and by the early afternoon, I had made it to almost 6 centimeters dilated. After about 6 hours of laboring without medication, my water broke naturally at 2:15 pm. My nurse was very adamant about having me lay on my left side so that they could monitor our daughter's heartbeat, which meant I was no longer able to move freely about the room and change position to cope with the surges. Despite my original plan to labor un-medicated, I asked for an epidural. The next 12 hours, I sat in my hospital bed peacefully and comfortably. The company of my husband, Brandon, his step mother, Nora, and my best friend, Aubrey, is truly what got me through my labor.

On April 13, 2019, at 2:05am a butterfly emerged.

She was 7 pounds, 14 ounces, 20 inches long and the most beautiful baby I had ever laid my eyes on. My heart dropped when I realized that she wasn't crying and I frantically started questioning why. The amount of time that passed before I received an answer seemed like an eternity. I will never forget the pain I felt, both physically and emotionally, as my doctor stitched up my 2nd degree tear and I watched a team of four nurses and a doctor try to resuscitate our daughter. I watched the color drain from my husband's face and thought for sure that we had lost her. After over an hour, I got a glimpse of her for a fleeting moment before she was rushed away to the Neonatal Intensive Care Unit (NICU).

The first day was a blur. I had no idea how she was doing. I hadn't held her. I had hardly gotten a look at her. All I knew was that her little lungs were full of fluid at birth and she had developed pneumonia. What should have been a two-day hospital stay turned into a nine-day stay as our daughter was put on antibiotics to fight the illness.

On April 15, 2019, at 10:07 am, I held our daughter for the first time. I stripped down to my nursing bra and mesh underwear and let the NICU nurses place my entire world on my chest. She had more wires than I could count attached to various parts of her body, a breathing tube in her nose and a feeding tube down her throat. I took note of them but not for more than a minute before I was flooded with joy. She was a cherub. On her face sat the sweetest little pair of lips and button nose and on her head was the thickest, darkest hair I had ever seen on a newborn. I couldn't take my eyes off of her. I stroked her hair and whispered to her countless times *"I love you so much Aubrey."* I can't remember exactly how long I sat there with her, but however long it was, did not feel long enough. Her skin was so soft and sweet-smelling and though she was but a day old, she held her head up so well to look at me. Did she know how long I had been waiting to meet her? Surely she did, she had been waiting to meet me too. There had been times in my life before where I struggled to find purpose... my purpose... but at that moment it became oh so clear. She was my purpose.

Later that afternoon, we attempted to breastfeed for the first time. Of course, it had been a couple of days since Aubrey was born and we didn't get to spend as much time together as most new moms and healthy babies do so it took a few tries to get it right. By the early evening, we had finally succeeded at getting her to latch. What an incredible flood of emotions. I remember feeling so relieved and overjoyed; I was no longer afraid that we wouldn't bond. I no longer felt this great disconnect from her. As strange as it sounds, until that moment I had only felt like *a mother* but as soon as she latched on... I was *her mother.*

For the rest of our hospital stay, I visited the NICU every three hours or whenever she woke up, whichever happened first. Though I was still sore and frankly sleep-deprived, I cherished every moment spent in that NICU nursing her. Every time she latched, I felt a wave of peace, comfort and warmth spread throughout my entire body. There was no place I would have rather been, except maybe at home curled up on the couch with her.

The moments between NICU visits were hard. I felt the dark cloud of postpartum depression rapidly forming over my head. I blamed myself for how she entered the world and felt guilty, like I had failed her. If not for my best friend, Aubrey, being there to remind me how strong and intuitive I was, I may not have stayed sane for our 9-day hospital stay. She praised me at the smallest moments. Like when I realized using the bathroom before pumping helped to reduce the postpartum contractions I was experiencing. Or when I told her I felt the impending depression, she told me how proud she was of me listening to my body and acknowledging what I was feeling instead of ignoring it. I had hoped that when we were finally released and able to create our own routine at home that things would get much easier.

The day we went home happened so fast, almost faster than the day she arrived. The NICU staff rushed to give us as much information as possible on how to care for her when we got home, but honestly, I can't remember any of it now. We fitted her into the car seat and were escorted out by one of the nurses. My husband drove calmly and carefully as I sat next to Aubrey in the back seat; we played classic rock the entire way and I sang her every song.

Like any other new, young family, the adjustment period was a little shaky. Even more so for us because we really didn't have a solid support system. My family was states away in Florida and though Brandon's family was close, they all always seemed too busy or just plain uninterested in helping. The only thing that helped me stay sane was the bond that was created between Aubrey and me by breastfeeding. Late at night when the room was dark and cool and the world was silent all the troubles of the day melted away. I would rock her and hum softly as she suckled, eyes closed and heartbeat steady. This was home, not a place but a feeling, a moment. Of all the things I had to be unsure about in this new role I played, I felt sure that I was providing the proper nourishment for my growing girl.

On April 24, 2019, Aubrey had her first doctor's visit outside of the hospital. This was our family's first time meeting her pediatrician, but she was recommended to us by my gynecologist, as well as some of the nurses from the office. I trusted their word because of the many things I had become responsible for, I didn't have the time or energy to look into a pediatrician on my own. No one ever tells you the things a breastfeeding mom should look for in a pediatrician for their child but, you live and learn.

Upon arrival, we were greeted by a very friendly staff of nurses who couldn't stop gushing over her long dark hair and golden skin tone. "A real-life baby doll," is how they described her; it wasn't the first time we had heard that and certainly wouldn't be the last. Aubrey was the picture of good health. Despite her stay in the NICU, she looked and acted like a remarkably healthy baby. Her doctor had absolutely no concerns, but did ask us a few times if I was sure that I wanted to breastfeed and offered us some samples of formula. There wasn't a doubt in my mind; I thanked her for the offer, but kindly declined. I didn't even want the thought of formula tempting me to stray away from breastfeeding. I knew there was nothing wrong with formula, but in my mind and heart, breastmilk was the best thing for my baby.

Nothing could beat the bond we shared, I wasn't going to let *anyone* break that.

May 2019

Motherhood and everything that came with it was relatively easy for me. I loved watching Aubrey learn, grow and develop new skills every day. There is just something so sublime about watching your child grow from a brand new soul depending on you for everything to a little person with their own personality, feelings and opinions. There was never a doubt in my mind that this is what I was meant to do. I felt myself transform, spiritually, from the Maiden to the Mother and I was really trying to enjoy every moment of finding myself in this new identity. It certainly didn't come without struggle, though. Having already been someone who previously suffered from depression and post-traumatic stress disorder, I was at a higher risk for developing postpartum depression than the majority of the population. That dark cloud I felt while we were still in the hospital continued to loom. Most days I felt fine, but just that. Fine.

In those first few months, I don't ever remember one day where I felt happy all day. I found little moments in each day that made me smile or laugh. Like the first time Aubrey held her head up or when she peed on me while I was changing her diaper. I always felt especially blissful while nursing her, that was something I was sure would never change. But the days always felt so long. I remember counting down the hours until my husband would be home from work, that was the only way I was able to stay sane. I was really struggling with the lack of sleep. Aubrey was a horrible sleeper. She would only nap for at most 20 minutes, unless she was being held, and even then I would get lucky to have her sleep for 45 minutes. Regrettable, I would lay with her on the couch during her nap times. I placed her high on my chest and propped us up with pillows, placing them under my arms and behind my head. I knew this was dangerous, but I was desperate for sleep and I couldn't figure out any other way to get it.

On top of the fact that she didn't sleep well, Aubrey was terribly colicky. She would scream for hours on end with almost no way to console her. I would rock her, bounce her, sing to her, swaddle her. I tried so many different things and nothing seemed to help. I remember staying with my brother-in-law's girlfriend for a week after Aubrey's first checkup. It was comforting to have the help especially because Brandon had to go right back to work but she said things to me like "Are you sure your milk isn't drying up?", "Maybe your milk isn't thick enough." "You know, WIC gives formula for free, why don't you just formula feed?" No matter how many times I told her I was determined to breastfeed, she still had unsolicited "advice" to give me about my choice. Every word she spoke against me breastfeeding just felt like a stab at my already fragile mental state. Why couldn't she understand that nursing was the only thing that helped me keep pushing. Aubrey and I had such an incredible breastfeeding relationship and for that, I was eternally grateful.

My confidence in our breastfeeding relationship was only strengthened at the beginning of her 2-month well-visit. I received confirmation from her pediatrician that our papillon was still growing on her growth curve, weighing in at 10 pounds 11 ounces, and that she looked healthy and happy. At the end of our appointment, I was asked if I had any concerns. I mentioned the fact that she was an awful sleeper and was almost always crying. Her pediatrician's solution was to give her formula. Despite the fact that I had already been told that she was gaining weight properly, I was advised to give her formula. I couldn't figure out why her doctor would even suggest that especially since I had already expressed that my goal was to exclusively breastfeed for at least two years. I reminded her of this, in case she had forgotten. She insisted that "formula will help her sleep" and offered me a few sample cans again. Once more, I politely declined and we were on our way home. I can recall being very frustrated that day and going home determined to find a solution to her sleep patterns. I couldn't shake the feeling that her pediatrician gave me towards the end of the appointment. Why had she offered me formula not once, but twice, both for reasons outside of lack of weight gain. That was the only reason I could justify supplementing with formula, but even then only after I had run out of frozen breastmilk.

Over the next few weeks, I started to notice that Aubrey was not only having problems sleeping but issues with spitting up as well. After nearly every nursing session, she would spit up what seemed like at least one to two ounces... Which at first blush does not seem like much, but to a breastfeeding baby it could be an entire feeding. I tried everything I could before calling doctor. I would burp her frequently throughout a feeding, sat her up for 30 minutes after nursing, I even tried gas drops. Nothing seemed to be working and I was running out of ideas. As a last resort, I called her doctor and her suggestion was... Formula. She told me that I was feeding her too often and that formula is thicker so it would stay in her stomach better. She advised me to only feed her every three to four hours asopposed to every two to two and a half hour as I had been. This didn't make any sense to me. I thought to myself, "If she's hungry, shouldn't I feed her?", "Even if she isn't hungry, shouldn't I still encourage her to latch? I'm her safe place and I want to continue to be her safe place." So, just as every time before, I politely thanked her for her input, but disregarded what she said. Maybe our papillon was just going through a phase that would end in a few months. Maybe her tiny newborn stomach was still maturing and I needed to give her time. So I gave her time.

Through her next two months of life, we endured sleepless nights that seemed far worse than what most new parents are told to expect and the spitting up only seemed to be getting worse. Despite the little voice in my head telling me that something was wrong, we just kept pushing on because she was otherwise such a happy and smart baby. She hit every milestone, and then some, early and was always laughing and smiling so I thought, "Maybe this is just how my baby is and eventually she'll grow out of it. She has to sleep at some point... she can't spit up forever." I never really noticed any lack of wet diapers or other of dehydration, but I guess in hindsight, I wasn't really looking for them.

I tried my best to cope with the lack of sleep until it was finally too much. I can't remember the exact day I reached my breaking point, but I remember exactly what happened. It was going on 6 hours and Aubrey hadn't fallen asleep for a nap yet. I had rocked and bounced and sang to her for hours and was slowly losing my mind. I remember eventually putting her down in her bassinet and running to hide in the bathroom.

With the room around me spinning and my head pounding, I made a post in a Facebook support group desperately asking for help. My crying turned into screams as the hair on my head was met with a grip almost tight enough to rip every strand out and Lord knows I wanted to. I was terrified that I was going to hurt Aubrey or myself and I was very seriously contemplating calling 9-11. The only thing that was holding me back was the fear of them taking her away from me. I sobbed and screamed for what felt like an eternity, all while listening to my daughter scream from the other room. I didn't know who to call or what to do. It felt like the four walls surrounding me were simultaneously swallowing and crushing me.

I can't remember for certain how long I was in that room before I finally brought myself out of the panic attack but once I did, I left the bathroom with a mission. I packed the diaper bag with a change of outfit for Aubrey, a few burp cloths, some snacks and water for myself and a large blanket. I brought the bag and my baby-wearing wrap upstairs, picked my daughter up from the bassinet and embraced her snuggly against my chest before securing her into the wrap. With her close to me and the diaper bag on my back, I put the leash on our dog and set out for the park down the street. I needed air. I had been cooped up for too long... we both had. The moment the wind met my face, I felt relief. I inhaled as deeply as I could and took a moment to collect my thoughts. We spent a few hours at the park that day and when we got home, she finally slept. That was the day I decided that sleep training would benefit our family. I was done with the sleepless nights and I didn't know if I would survive another breakdown like that one.

After only a week my daughter started sleeping through the night, 12 hours straight! Every parent's dream, right? I was catching up on all the sleep I had lost the months prior and I felt much more mentally and emotionally stable. I was so sure we had made the right choice and I felt proud of myself for doing it. For two months, I bragged to family and friends about how my daughter no longer woke up in the middle of the night. Finally, one of the two problems we had been dealing with was solved. I'll never forget the little yawn, stretch and smile she gave me when I went to wake her up every morning. Some mornings, it was harder to wake her up than others. In hindsight, it became slightly more difficult with each passing day. She was sleeping soundly though, so maybe she just wasn't a morning person. Still, like every other warning sign, I pushed aside the little voice in my head because otherwise Aubrey was a happy, sassy, loving baby. *That much would never change.*

August 2019

As time passed, I watched Aubrey's skills really take off. It seemed like every day she learned to do something new. I was so amazed by her and everyone around us seemed to be too. No one really noticed anything "off" about her and neither did I until one of my close friends asked if she could buy Aubrey some clothing and wanted to know what size she was. At four months old I was just realizing that Aubrey was still swimming in her 0-3-month size clothing. This was a little odd to me because one of the things that other parents always commented on is how fast children grow. It didn't seem to me that Aubrey had really grown much physically but mentally she was leaps and bounds beyond her peers. Either way, her four-month well-visit was just a few days away, so I tried to ease my mind until then.

Just as our previous appointments, this one started with the staff cooing over how beautiful and alert Aubrey was. The nurse called us to the back and asked me to undress Aubrey so that she could be weighed. I brought my fussy baby over to the scale and waited anxiously for the numbers to stop blinking. When they did my heart dropped and everything around me started moving in slow motion. I started to dissociate and in the background, I heard the nurse whisper *"10 pounds, 10 ounces."* How could this be? What was I doing wrong? She gently said, "Okay, the doctor will be right with you." and quietly left the room. I turned to my husband.

"She hasn't gained any weight." He looked at me confused. "Are you sure? Maybe it's just the scale." Just as he said that the nurse came back in. "Can I just have you put her on the scale one more time?" "Sure," I said as I slowly stood back up and carried Aubrey to the scale, reluctantly placing her on it. It seemed that the numbers blinked for far longer this time. 10 pounds 8 ounces. I felt the color from my face drain and tried not to make eye contact with the nurse as she left the room, this time without saying anything. "It's okay babe. It's going to be okay." Brandon tried to comfort me, but I could tell he didn't know what to say. I was speechless... emotionless... numb.

"Okay mom, we're going to try her on this other scale, could you bring her to this room?" the nurse said peeking into the room. Brandon and I made our way to the room across the hall, but it felt like we were walking straight into our graves. I felt dead inside and I knew my face was paler than it had ever been. While the rest of me was numb, my thoughts were racing. I was trying to figure out how I could have let this happen. My thoughts were abruptly interrupted by the nurse's voice. "Okay, you guys can go ahead back to the other room," she said as Brandon and I turned to leave.

"What did it say?" I asked, not realizing that I had completely separated myself from reality for a moment. "10 pounds, 8 ounces." He was trying not to let on that he was concerned, but I could tell that he was. He would have to be crazy not to be concerned. After a few minutes, Aubrey's pediatrician came into the room and began giving us the 5th degree. "When did you notice that she wasn't gaining weight? Why didn't you bring her in?" she asked, almost as if she was accusing us of doing this on purpose.

"I-I don't know... I don't weigh her at home so I didn't notice. She's always so happy and she's hitting all of her milestones, I just... I wasn't paying attention." I was trying to hold back my tears. I was confused, concerned, and hurt all at the same time. Why was she making me feel like this was all my fault? Then again, wasn't it? "Okay, so what you will have to do now is give her 6 ounces of formula every 4 hours."

"Wait, but I'm breastfeeding," I couldn't believe, yet again, she was pushing formula. In this new, fragile state it was hard not to let my emotions drive me.

"Well, your milk isn't enough, that's why she's lost weight."

"Can't I just continue to nurse her and give her some of my frozen milk after each session until she gains the weight back?"

"You probably don't have enough." Why would she assume this?

"I have over 250 ounces. I think that's plenty." At this point, I was annoyed. I couldn't understand why the doctor was insisting that I stop breastfeeding and use formula before allowing me to supplement with my frozen milk. It couldn't make sense of it.

"Well let's just use the formula first and then if you want to go back to breastfeeding after she gains weight again then you can."

"I don't want to stop breastfeeding though."

"Yeah, but you see the problem is she hasn't gain any weight and she's actually lost weight. So use this formula and then come back in a week, so we can weigh her again." She handed us a bag full of large cans of formula.

"I still don't understand why I can't just supplement with my milk when I have so much of it." I kept pressing on but the doctor wasn't budging. Eventually, I took the formula from her just so that we

21

could leave.

On the way home, I tried to hide the tears racing down my face from Brandon. I didn't want him to know how defeated and worthless I felt, but I know he could feel it.

"It'll be okay, babe. We'll just use your milk first and then go from there. We don't have to use the formula."

I couldn't even talk. All I could think about was the fact that my daughter wasn't gaining weight and I never noticed. I couldn't stop blaming myself. How awful of a mother does someone have to be to not notice that their infant isn't gaining weight? I was just so confused and scared. My mind was racing and I remember feeling dizzy and hot. The only thing I wanted to do was pull Aubrey out of the car seat and hold her and never let her go. I wanted her to know how sorry I was for failing her as badly as I had. How do you explain to your four-month-old that you're sorry? How do you apologize in a way that they understand? Did she even know how I had hurt her? When she looks at me I see the pure unconditional love that she has for me but I didn't feel deserving of it in that moment.

When we finally got home, I tossed the bag of formula on the dining room table and ran downstairs to lock myself in the bathroom. I needed a good cry. The silent, gut wrenching kind. I needed to allow myself to feel what I was feeling before I could make a game plan on how to fix the problem. The pediatrician was clearly not going to be helpful and I had every intention of finding a new one anyway. For what seemed like hours, I let myself feel broken, helpless and lost, then collected myself to create a plan of action.

After Aubrey was down for her nap, I told Brandon how I wanted to tackle the issue.

"I think that the best way to do this is nurse her more often and then top every feeding off with 2 oz. of my milk but only if she doesn't seem satisfied after nursing."

"Okay, if that's what you want to do then that's what we'll do."

So we did, and for just a few days things seemed to be getting better. Aubrey wasn't as fussy after feedings and I was even noticing an increase in her diaper count. Until suddenly things took a dramatic turn for the worst.

On August 14th, I noticed that my urine was incredibly orange. Almost neon orange, which led me to believe I was extremely dehydrated. So I drank as much water and electrolyte replacing fluids as I could. Then two days later I noticed that my stool was clay colored and of course that sent me into a panic. As I researched my symptoms I settled on Hepatitis A and tried to make an appointment to see my primary care doctor but the only opening was a few days out so I waited anxiously.

On the evening of August 17th, I tried to fall asleep but was kept awake by unbearable pain that I thought was coming from my liver. I held out as long as I could but by midnight I could hardly breathe so I called my step-father-in-law to take me to the hospital. After 7 hours in the emergency department, several rounds of blood work and cat scans I had a diagnosis. Gallstones. The stones and my gallbladder would have to be removed but before that happened I was in the hospital for 3 days.

Those 3 days were absolute torture. I tried to latch Aubrey as much as possible but often times she would get fussy and Brandon kept forgetting the pumped milk. I felt like I was starving our sweet girl. On top of the fact that she wasn't napping well and when I pumped I wasn't getting as much as I usually did which of course was incredibly discouraging. Still, I pressed on. I knew if I could just get better, leave the hospital and find a little calmer in my environment that Aubrey and I would be able to get back on track. I continued to latch her at least twice a day throughout my hospital stay and kept her in the room with me except for when Brandon took her home at night so that she could sleep comfortably in her crib.

The day after having my surgery, Aubrey had her follow up appointment with the pediatrician. I was a ball of nerves but I knew that no matter what happened I was going to be leaving the practice and requesting all of Aubrey's paperwork. The waiting room was quiet and it felt like we were waiting to be assigned a grave. It was colder than usual and the faces behind the desk didn't feel as welcoming.

We waited in our usual room and much quicker than we were used to, the nurse came in to weigh Aubrey. She had gained a few ounces in about a week. Almost immediately after the nurse left Aubrey's pediatrician came in.

"So she's only gained a few ounces. Are you giving her the formula?"

I could feel the blood travel up my face and out the crown of my head.

"No." I was straight faced, trying my hardest to contain the fuming mess of emotions building up within me.

"Why not?" I felt a guilt trip coming.

"I have plenty of breastmilk at home and there's absolutely no reason why I shouldn't be able to use it." "Yeah but you see, she still hasn't gained much weight. I mean how much breastmilk are you giving her? You should be given her 6 oz. every 4 hours"

"After nursing her? That's just too much, she doesn't even take 4 oz. in one sitting, much less after nursing."

"You shouldn't be breastfeeding her at all. I'm going to send you to the emergency room because it's extremely concerning that she isn't gaining weight and you haven't been feeding her."

"That doesn't make any sense. I just told you what we've been doing. I *am* feeding her just not the way you want me to and you know what we're going to be seeing another doctor anyway so I would like all of her records and paperwork."

"That's fine. Who is the new pediatrician? I'll just fax the paperwork."

"No I would like physical copies of her paperwork, please." I could tell that now she was getting annoyed with me. She wasn't the best at hiding emotion from her face and even if she were, her cold tone of voice said all I needed to know.

"Who is her new pediatrician?"

"I don't have to disclose that information to you. I would appreciate her records in my hands before I leave this office."

"You know you're really making this difficult. What is *wrong* with you?" Never in my life had I been spoken to like that by a healthcare professional. It took everything in my power not to use every unsavory word I knew.

"Excuse me? How dare you speak to the parent of one of your patients like that. I am her mother and I am asking for her medical records. I have a right to them. I do not have to disclose any information to you and especially not who her new pediatrician is."

With that she put her tail between her legs and told me she would provide me with the paperwork I asked for, but not before telling me that I needed to take Aubrey over to the Emergency Department. That much I could agree to because, though I was livid with the doctor, my concern for Aubrey's health was more important.

August 2019 Part II

Before we drove over to the Emergency Department, we sat in the car so that I could cry again. This time it was different. Not the silent kind of crying but the kind that's so loud and powerful that you have trouble catching your breath. Just when I thought things couldn't have been any worse than they were the past week, I was proven wrong. The last thing I wanted to do was spend an indefinite amount of time at the hospital with our daughter but I knew that we needed to figure out what was going on.

The Emergency Department knew we were coming and upon arrival took us back to one of the triage rooms to begin running tests. We arrived a little after 10 am and somewhere around 5 pm tests were done and they found nothing wrong with her. This was both a good and bad thing. Nothing was wrong with her heart and all her bloodwork came back normal but that meant I was now to blame for her lack of weight gain. My breast milk was to blame.

I explained to the doctors my theory. That I didn't realize how sick I was and how my gallbladder issues were causing me to become dehydrated which in turn caused my milk supply to drop. The doctors wanted to make sure that she was able to retain the fluids she was taking in so we were admitted to the pediatric floor for monitoring. No one could tell us how long we would be there but I had a feeling it would be our new home for a while.

The nurses were very polite and, like everyone who has met Aubrey, wouldn't stop cooing over how beautiful and alert she was. Aubrey was responsive to their faces, smiling and laughing at the attention. In this moment, Aubrey taught me something. No matter how bad your situation might seem, there is beauty to be found somewhere. I am eternally grateful for that.

We spent the next four days getting to know the nurses from each shift and the doctors on call. Every passing minute felt like days and they were all starting to blur together. The staff wanted to make sure that Aubrey could retain what she took in so everything had to be documented. Every ounce going in needed to be recorded, which meant they wouldn't let me breastfeed. I had to pump and bottle feed her.

"So here's the sheet. Every time you or someone on staff feeds her it needs to be written down. The amount and the time." The day shift nurse handed me a sheet of paper and a pencil.

"Okay, I can do that." I remember feeling overwhelmed but determined to do whatever I had to in order to get us out of the hospital as soon as possible.

"Same with diapers. Write the time and if it was wet or dirty. One of the nurses will weigh them though so put them in the grey tub on the counter." she said pointing to the counter by the door. I was having trouble focusing. She went on to give me some more information but my thoughts were elsewhere.

Did they think we were neglecting Aubrey? Why couldn't I breastfeed her? Surely the stress of being here on top of just having had surgery will cause my supply to drop. How long will we be here?

"Okay, we'll leave you guys to get settled." the nurse turned to walk out the door, just before she left I called out to her. "Oh wait! Is there any update on me getting a breast pump? I haven't pumped since 10 this morning and I'm supposed to pump every 3 hours."

"Oh yes. I'll check on that for you." She closed the door behind her. I looked over at Aubrey in the hospital crib. It was asylum white and sides were so high that it looked like a baby jail cell. It was supposed to keep her safe but it felt more like a punishment. Why was she being punished for something that was my fault? I was supposed to be the one keeping her safe. Yet through the colorless confinement Aubrey was happy, unassuming and unaware of the danger these healthcare professionals thought she was in.

Not long after the nurse left, a group of doctors and interns came in to introduce themselves, tell us the game plan and ask if we had any questions.

"So basically we'll record everything she takes in. Every morning we'll weigh her to see how much she's gained since the morning before. We'll also weigh every diaper as well. We want to make sure that your milk supply is coming back in too so we'll monitor that to make sure you're producing the same amount that she's taking in." The intern doctor repeated everything the nurses told me and then gave me space to ask questions or address any concerns. He clearly was the one who needed to be asking questions. I was a novice at breastfeeding, but even I knew that pumping is never a good indication of how much milk someone is producing.

"I just have concerns about the pumping part. I don't always respond well to pumping. Sometimes I pump an ounce sometimes I pump five ounces. Pumping really isn't a good indication of supply..." I trailed off. These doctors didn't understand and I could tell by the looks on their faces. Why don't they train pediatric doctors to know at least the basics of breastfeeding? I'm sure that babies who are nursing aren't typically in the hospital like this but if I was, there had to be other parents with children in the hospital for the same reason at some point in history. I couldn't possibly have been the first. Which made me think, *'how many other parents were told they had a low milk supply based solely off of what they were pumping?'* This didn't seem fair, surely not every parent was as educated about breastfeeding as I felt I was.

"Well, we can worry about that when the time comes. If you're not producing enough we'll just go to formula." There was word again. *Formula.* I've always known that formula is an option for parents who can't or don't want to breastfeed and I support that, but I *can* and I *do* want to breastfeed so why on earth is it being pushed on me every time I turn around? I sighed and gave up on trying to give any sort of thought out response.

"Well, if you have no other questions then we'll leave you guys to finish settling."

"Nope, I think that's it." I turned to hide my face. Couldn't anyone see how stressed I was? Don't they know how stress can impact one's milk supply? All I wanted was to feel that same bond I had when we first started breastfeeding. The closeness, the feeling that I was the only one who could nourish her, the feeling that she needed me. Being here at the hospital made me feel the exact opposite. I felt useless and unwanted. Why would she want to breastfeed when all these nurses were giving her bottles and she didn't have to work for them? I never did move past that feeling.

About a day into our stay, I was contacted by my

30

mother-in-law. I didn't want to tell her what was happening but when she started asking questions I just couldn't lie to her. It did seem like she had our best interest at heart but some of the things she said were more hurtful than I think she realized.

"Well, it sounds like they're just concerned about your milk not having enough calories for her, which is probably the problem. I'll reach out to a family friend who had problems with her supply and see what supplement she recommends." She was always so quick to offer help, one of her best qualities. She came to the hospital a few days later with a vitamin supplement that was supposed to help my supply and included an herb called Fenugreek. At that point, I was willing to try just about anything to bring my supply back up just so that the doctors would let us go sooner.

I was diligent throughout the course of our hospital stay. If they gave Aubrey a bottle then I was up pumping at the exact same time, day and night. I always asked them to wake me up but they never did. They thought they were doing me a favor by letting me sleep, but what they were really doing was putting my milk supply (and my sanity) at risk. I genuinely could not wrap my head around the fact that these healthcare professionals seemed to be absolutely clueless when it came to how milk production worked. Honestly, they seemed clueless about how babies worked in general.

They were always saying things like "She's sucking her thumb, she must be hungry," when in reality Aubrey would suck her thumb to soothe herself if she was tired, bored, upset, uncomfortable and so many reasons other than being hungry (to this day she still does.) They shoved a bottle in her mouth every time she

31

cried and always tried to make her finish the entire thing even when she was visibly full. Then when she spat up they blamed it on my breastmilk saying that it was "too thin." None if it made any sense to me and more than anything it was incredibly stressful and demeaning. I felt like a terrible and inadequate mother. Though at this point, one would have thought I had gotten used to that feeling.

Eventually, when the hospital staff was satisfied that Aubrey was able to retain weight after taking a bottle, they let me nurse. The moment she latched, I felt a wave of overwhelming relief and serenity. The hospital room and everyone in it ceased to exist, it was just Aubrey and me. I remember savoring that moment more than the first time she latched. It felt so special because for days I felt we were kept apart against our will. I was forced to sit in the corner and pump while someone else bonded with my daughter through feeding. I worried the entire time she wouldn't want to latch because she had developed a preference for the bottle nipple. But, we were, peacefully lounging as she gently suckled on my breast. Then, when I thought the moment couldn't possibly be more sublime, I heard one of the nurses speak to me.

"So, what do you think, would you like to see a lactation consultant?"

I looked up at her, my face absolutely beaming. That was the first time anyone had offered to bring a lactation consultant in and I certainly did not feel comfortable asking especially since they weren't even letting me nurse.

"Oh yes please, I would love that!" I replied. With enthusiasm, "Great! We'll call to have someone come up here before the end of the day." The nurse left with a smile. I looked up at Brandon and I could see the relief in his face.

Surely, watching me under so much stress was doing just the same to him. I brought Aubrey up to my shoulder to burp her when I noticed that she was done nursing and whispered in her ear, "We're going to get this figured out petit papillon." Her sweet cheeks were pressed up against my body and I listened to the subtle wave of her breath as she drifted off to sleep.

It wasn't long before the lactation consultant came in. She was a soft spoken woman, but very clearly enjoyed her job. She watched quietly as Aubrey nursed for a little while and then took a bottle. Afterwards, the lactation consultant wanted to take a look inside of her mouth. I watched a gloved finger maneuver about my daughter's cheeks, tongue and upper lip. The exam was fairly quick.

"Now, technically, I'm not supposed to give a formal diagnosis because I'm not an International Board Certified Lactation Consultant (IBCLC) but I went through all of this with my daughter. I'm pretty certain that Aubrey has a tongue tie." She handed Aubrey back to me and took the gloves off her hands before reaching into her pocket for a piece of paper and a pen.

"There's one doctor in the state who is well known for correcting oral ties. He worked with my daughter and I, and he's amazing so I'm going to write down his contact information. Just in case he doesn't take your insurance I'm also going to write down a backup doctor."

Though grateful for what seemed like the first real answer I had received since this whole ordeal started, I was a little overwhelmed. I had heard of a tongue tie before, but I supposed I didn't know as much about them as I thought because I never noticed anything wrong with Aubrey's tongue.

I smiled at the lactation consultant as she handed the paper to me. "Thank you so much. Really, you have no idea what we've been through and I finally feel like I'm being heard. I knew there was nothing wrong with my milk supply."

"You are welcome. Please try to call this doctor as soon as possible, you'll probably have to do physical therapy with her after the correction, but you should be able to go back to breastfeeding with no problem." She flashed a smile and gave me a hug before leaving the room.

"Do you feel better now that you've seen a lactation consultant?" Brandon came over to embrace Aubrey and me. I took a deep breath before responding.

"I really do. And I can't wait to get out of here tomorrow. I think I still want to see an IBCLC when we get home just to be sure, but I do feel relieved that it seems like we have somewhat of an answer now." In that breath, I felt the mom guilt being lifted from my shoulders and knew that there was still hope for us to meet the breastfeeding goal I had set.

September 2019

Being home felt so incredible. After living at a hospital for nearly two weeks, I was so happy to be back to somewhat normal. No more doctors monitoring me or Aubrey, no more having to worry about the nurses overfeeding her or not letting me breastfeed. I was once again in the comfort of my own home and even had a little extra help since my sister flew in from Florida to help us out while I recovered from gallbladder surgery.

I eventually got around to calling the doctor recommended by the lactation consultant in the hospital but when I spoke to the nurse on staff she informed me that they did not take the insurance we had. I was disappointed but decided that I would seek out an IBCLC. In the meantime, I came up with a plan on how to feed Aubrey until that could happen. She was still happily latching, so I let her as much as she wanted, that never changed. But, if I ever felt as though she was dissatisfied by the amount of milk she was getting I would top her feeding off with an ounce or two of pumped milk or formula. I knew that in any other circumstance this wouldn't be necessary, but Aubrey had a lot of weight to gain before she was back on the growth charts and I knew that, at the very least, I needed to supplement until that happened. Luckily she seemed satisfied by nursing most times. She would nurse for 20-30 minutes before unlatching herself, letting a little bit of milk dribble out of the corner of her sweet smile. I never did get tired of her sweet milky breath.

In the first few days that followed our return, I researched until all hours of the night looking for an

IBCLC who would be able to tell us for sure what the issue was with Aubrey nursing. After going through countless Facebook groups, google searches and twitter posts I found an IBCLC who serviced the greater Baltimore area. A difficult conversation with Brandon followed, as I discovered she didn't take insurance and it would cost us over $200 out-of-pocket. To me it was well worth it but it took some convincing because money was tight. He did give in eventually and I was able to schedule an appointment for the second week of that month.

My first impression of Katy was that she was sweet. She spoke fast and had a warm smile and most importantly she seemed knowledgeable. We spent the first hour of the consultation going over medical history for myself and Aubrey as any relevant family medical history. Once she had all the information she needed she wanted to weigh Aubrey and then watch her nurse. It didn't take long for her to notice that Aubrey was having trouble creating a proper suction on my breast. Katy also weighed Aubrey after she was done nursing which is how we discovered she didn't transfer much milk from the breast. In fact, she transferred less than an ounce, which was obviously not enough to satisfy her. There was that guilty feeling again. Had I not been supplementing enough when I gave her a bottle? I didn't realize she was taking so little in.

After review, she said, "So, Aubrey does have a tongue tie, but it's pretty minor so it shouldn't need to be corrected. I'll send you some exercises to do to help strengthen her jaw and things should start getting easier soon. I also want you to purchase a different supplement for your milk supply since the one you've been using with Fenugreek in it actually decreases milk supply in moms with Polycystic Ovarian Syndrome like you."

I responded, "It doesn't need to be corrected? The lactation consultant in the hospital recommended Doctor Marcus to correct it and she mentioned that she had similar issues with her daughter before her tongue tie was corrected."

"I'm not a huge fan of Doctor Marcus. You don't need to get it corrected, she just needs to strengthen her jaw." This all felt so off to me, but I was inclined to trust Katy because of all the great reviews I read about her, in addition to her board certification. So I decided to go with her word and hope the exercises she gave me would be enough to solve our breastfeeding issues. We said a quick goodbye and as soon as she left, I expressed my doubt to Brandon.

"I don't think that these exercises are going to make a difference. All the groups I'm in on Facebook say that tongue ties have to be corrected especially if you're having trouble nursing and that there really isn't such a thing as a minor oral tie."

"Well, do you want to look for a place to get it corrected then? I think we should at least do the exercises and then go from there."

I responded to Brandon saying, "I guess we can do the exercises." I was reluctant, but after spending over $200 to see Katy I thought I should at least give it a try. I followed Katy's instructions word for word for about a week before I emailed her with a new development.

To: Katy From: Kylia
Date: September 16, 2019 9:24:00 AM EST

Hi Katy,

I *think* things are going much better. I haven't had a chance to order the supplements yet but we didn't have to give Aubrey a bottle at all yesterday or the day before! She seemed totally satisfied after nursing and had 4-6 pretty heavy wet diapers and 1 dirty diaper each day.

Yesterday afternoon she started fussing towards the end of a nursing session though. She had already nursed on both sides for about 10 minutes each and then unlatched and looked around then latched back for about 30 seconds and then unlatched and started fussing. I thought maybe she was trying to get another let down but when I tried a little hand expression there was *definitely* milk flowing. (aka I drenched her face in milk). I tried to get her to latch back but she refused.

She's been doing this since yesterday afternoon (6 times total). I'm wondering if she's started doing this because she's done nursing? I'm just not used to her latching for such short sessions. All 6 times she nursed for less than 15 minutes' total. I appreciate any insight!

Warm Regards,

Kylia.

A few days later I got a response but Katy didn't answer my question or address my concern. The only thing she asked was how many times a day she was nursing. I responded by telling her roughly 6-8 times in 24 hours to which she responded,

"I would try to make sure she gets 8 feedings in a day, she really needs 8-10. That will help."

This still wasn't a clear answer for the very straightforward question I had asked but I did as she suggested and increased our nursing sessions. However, 5 days later I emailed her again with more questions.

To: Katy From: Kylia
Date: September 23, 2019 6:57:00 PM EST

Hi Katy,

So we upped the nursing sessions to about 10 times in 24 hours... I tried the supplements, they haven't helped. It actually seems like my supply has dropped again and we are back to giving her a bottle after just about every feeding (even at night which never happened before).

The exercises don't really seem to be working either as she is still chomping on my breast as opposed to sucking. I'm not sure where to go from here.

This was right around the time I started to regret not just looking for a provider to correct the tongue tie in the first place. I felt like Katy had really led me astray from my goals and hadn't taken the time to even address my concerns the way she should have. It was almost four days before I received an email back from her which was only more questions for me. She asked how much time Aubrey was spending on her tummy as well as if we were still doing bottles and how often I was pumping. Had she not read my email? I wasn't sure what tummy time had to do with anything. I suppose the pumping question was relevant but I had already mentioned that we were giving her bottles after nearly every feeding. I responded to her email almost immediately after I received it.

To: Katy From: Kylia
Date: September 27, 2019 5:51:00 AM EST

Hi Katy,
*   She's almost always on her tummy, she loves to roll. Bottles have been increased because she is so fussy while nursing and sometimes she doesn't even want to latch. I pump every 2 hours during the day and 3-4 at night. If I pump before nursing I get maybe an ounce, if I pump after nursing I get 2-5 oz.*

I waited a week without a response before I followed up. Now I was getting more than just frustrated. I was angry. I knew that I couldn't possibly be the only parent that Katy was working with but I also couldn't understand how she was not only leaving my questions unanswered when she did respond but also just not responding. Despite being as angry as I was, I tried to write my follow up email as politely as possible.

Hi Katy,

I'm feeling a little discouraged because as per your website and the conversation we had before you left my house, I was under the impression that you would be available for guidance as we try to get Aubrey back on track with exclusively nursing. However, since that day I don't feel that you have answered any of my questions and it has also taken quite some time to even get a response from you. I can't say that I am satisfied with the service you have provided since the initial consultation.

I understand that you are a busy lactation consultant with, I'm sure, a lot of moms who require your help. However, as one of those moms, I did think I would receive a little more help.

I have not nursed Aubrey for over a week now because she refuses to latch at all. I can't help but feel like if my questions had been answered by you, and in a timely manner, that we could have avoided this. So, now I'm not sure where to go from here.

I would really appreciate some guidance.
Thank You. Kylia

Even after sending that email, I still waited another 4 days before I received a response. She apologized and said her children were sick and then followed up with more questions about how much milk I was pumping and said I should start doing skin-to-skin to get her interested in latching again. After I responded to her email with the answers to her questions, I didn't hear back from her for a month. That response was only after I left a review on the Facebook and Google page for her business informing other parents of the experience I had. For an entire month I didn't hear a single word from her. I couldn't believe that even after she offered an apology and I expressed that I was willing to give her a second chance, she still did not address my concerns or answer my questions. Over the course of that month we did have some good news from Aubrey's new pediatrician who said that she was gaining weight beautifully and encouraged us to continue doing what we were doing. I was able to find a provider who corrected Aubrey's lip tie but told me that she didn't have a tongue tie. Which of course left me just as confused and with the lack of help I received from Katy I had to set out on my own, once again, to find answers.

I was a member of several parenting and breastfeeding Facebook groups at the time and decided to post asking for help. I explained what happened with Katy and the other provider and how we still were having trouble with nursing. Almost instantly at least ten other parents commented on my post recommending none other than Dr. Marcus. Just moments later. I received both a friend request and Facebook message from Dr. Marcus himself. He introduced himself to me, gave me his personal cell phone number and asked me to call him the following day so that I would have an opportunity to explain our situation a little better. This was the first time in months I actually felt like some progress would be made. By this point, Aubrey was still latching but not very often. I was glad to tell Dr. Marcus everything that we had experienced and after I was done he had one of his nurses make an appointment for a consultation at the beginning of December. So all I had to do was keep Aubrey interested in latching for the next month.

November 2019

November was a bit of a break from the mayhem of the past few months but that doesn't mean it was easy by any means. I tried everything I possibly could to keep Aubrey interested in latching, but it was difficult because I was getting constant clogged milk ducts. I was in an incredible amount of pain and it made nursing no longer the blissful experience it used to be. Yet I was still as determined as ever. I took baths with Aubrey, gave her bottles topless and close to my breast, I even tried to "trick" her by touching her face with the bottle nipple before swiftly putting my breast in her mouth. Sometimes my tricks worked and other times they didn't but I never gave up.

When Thanksgiving finally came around it was nice to be surrounded by family. With my parents and siblings in town, some family friends and Brandon's dad and step-mom, it was a full house. We spent the day cooking, laughing and just enjoying each other's company. I was happy to let others give Aubrey her bottles because to be honest, all the time I was spending so close to her was causing me to feel touched out. Parents aren't supposed to get tired of cuddling their babies, but I was starting to dread having to be around Aubrey. I didn't feel like my body belonged to me anymore, I was a stranger in it. I couldn't remember the last time I recognized myself when I looked in the mirror. Was this normal? Did other parents ever feel the same way? Surely, I couldn't be the only one. I loved Aubrey more than anyone or thing in the world, but some days were just so stressful and I felt so guilty for not wanting to be around her. Society taught me that my baby comes first and my feelings don't matter. I wasn't allowed to want a break or to need space and that felt so consuming... so suffocating. I just needed to breathe and I rarely ever got the chance to.

I got so many questions from my family and friends that day. "Are you still breastfeeding?", "Why aren't you giving her formula?", "She was fussing after her bottle, should I just give her more?" I know that everyone was just curious and trying to help, but it did feel like my ability to be a mother was being questioned. Like no one trusted me when I said she wasn't hungry after a 4 oz. bottle or just because she was crying didn't mean she wanted more. Though the company was much needed, it made me realize how much this whole situation had really taken a toll on my confidence as a mother. I don't think I had taken note of it before that day.

January 2020

Between Thanksgiving and the day, we went to see Dr. Marcus, Aubrey had stopped latching completely. Every single time I tried to offer my breasts, she would scream at the top of her lungs and push away from me. No amount of skin to skin or "tricking her" or even putting syrup on my nipple made her want to latch on. I didn't want to give up though. I held on to hope that after getting her tongue tie corrected and seeing a speech therapist, as recommended by Dr. Marcus, that she would gain interest again.

Unfortunately, the day of our consultation we were almost 30 minutes late. Dr. Marcus was still able to see us and confirm her tongue tie but he didn't have time to correct it before his next appointment. So we waited another month before finally having it corrected just after the New Year. I remember the day like it was yesterday, I felt nervous, but relieved. I knew that the correction would be painful for Aubrey but I knew in the long run she would benefit from it. And, I still had hope that she would latch again.

Brandon, Aubrey and I sat anxiously in the waiting room to be called in. Everything seemed to be moving much faster around me as I drifted through my thoughts. I hoped that she wouldn't resent me for having this done. I hoped that she was still too young to remember. The one thing that I was holding on to was how gentle and kind Dr. Marcus was. He made me feel like, despite the discomfort Aubrey would experience, it was well worth it to prevent several years of problems like speech impediments, chronic muscle tension, pain and so much more.

When we were finally called in Dr. Marcus took time to explain the procedure to us again and gave us an opportunity to ask questions. At that point, I just wanted to get it done and over with. He asked, "Would you like to stay in the room during this procedure?" I immediately said no and walked out. I couldn't even handle watching Aubrey cry from getting her vaccinations, let alone a procedure she should have had done months ago. I was relieved to let Brandon stay with her and sit in the waiting room until they were done.

Less than 2 minutes later, Brandon walked out into the waiting room with Aubrey. She was visibly upset, but as soon as she was in my arms she instantly melted and calmed down. I was so happy that even though we hadn't nursed in a while, I was still a source of comfort for her.

Dr. Marcus took us back to a separate waiting room to feed her. He said that usually nursing or taking a bottle immediately after the procedure helped the babies to settle. I waited until he walked out to try to get her to latch but when it didn't happen right away I, surprisingly, wasn't as upset as I had been in the weeks prior. I knew that she had just been through something painful and still didn't realize that she would now be able to extract milk from my breast properly. I settled on giving her a bottle and then we went home.

In the weeks that followed, we saw a Speech Language Pathologist. She helped us work with Aubrey on retraining her how to use her tongue properly. I definitely saw a difference in the mobility of her tongue almost instantly and just the same, I noticed she wasn't dribbling when she took her bottle. Day in and day out, I did what I could to help her regain interest in nursing. All the same tricks I tried before her tongue tie was correct with a few new ones.

One of my favorite ones to try was letting her watch me hand express milk. She was getting to the age where she was so curious about everything and this was something that always peaked her interest. So often she would watch the milk flow from my nipple and give it a soft kiss or even open her mouth a bit to taste the milk. This happened enough times to make me feel like soon, she would latch again. So I pushed as long and hard as I could.

March 2020

As I said in the prologue, this is a story I started writing before I knew how it would end. March of 2020 was when our family packed up and moved from Maryland to Georgia in the midst of a global pandemic – COVIDD 19. The chaos of packing up the house, saying our goodbyes and flying across several states was so stressful. I couldn't fathom attempting to keep up with pumping every 3 hours on top of trying to get Aubrey to latch again. Slowly, but surely, my milk supply started to dwindle away as I dropped pumping sessions because they became more and more of an inconvenience.

Aubrey started walking, which made sitting down with her to offer my breast nearly impossible. Through everything we had experienced, it pained me to wave the white flag, but it was clear that we had come to the end of our journey.

A few days before we moved, I washed out all of my pump parts and bottles and packed them away with my pump and milk storage bags. My cheeks were met with salty wet pearls as I taped the box up and labeled it "breastfeeding supplies". Every memory of us nursing came flooding back all at once and I felt a lump growing in my throat as more tears streamed down my face.

What we put up with didn't seem fair. I felt like I had been robbed of something I waited my entire life to experience.

The day I packed those supplies away was the day that made me 100% confident in my decision to write a book. I had decided months ago, to start documenting our experience and I was almost certain I wanted to get it published, but the way I felt in that moment made me more sure than I had ever been. I knew I never wanted another parent to have to go through what we did. Surely, I wasn't the first and I knew I wouldn't be the last, but if I could help even one parent avoid having a similar experience then I was certainly going to try.

Epilogue

There were so many things that served as a catalyst for the failure of our breastfeeding journey. Looking back, it could have all been avoided, but let's start with the beginning, the day Aubrey was born.

One of the tell-signs of a tongue tie is a cupped tongue when crying. All of the pictures of Aubrey from when she was in the NICU show a very visible cupped tongue. Why did none of the nurses notice this? Were they not trained to identify warning signs of an oral tie? And if not, why? Though the NICU nurses were the least of my concerns at that point and even now.

When a new parent visits the pediatrician with their child for the first time after they are born, why is formula immediately offered? Before I even had the opportunity to express how committed I was to breastfeeding, formula was pushed on me. And, at every inconvenience, the answer was just the same. Had our pediatrician been knowledgeable in the slightest on oral ties, she would have picked up on the issues we were having. Aubrey's trouble sleeping, her constant spitting up, and finally her lack of weight gain. The latter of, which, could have been prevented had any of the former problems been caught. What truly should have happened was a much simpler answer. A referral to a specialist, someone like, or maybe even, Dr. Marcus.

I'll admit supplementing was incredibly important after we learned that Aubrey was not gaining weight. What I never understood was the lack of support behind my desire to supplement with my pumped milk. Even more so, why didn't the pediatrician make sure to mention that no matter what I used to supplement, I needed to pump every time I gave Aubrey a bottle otherwise I would begin to lose my milk supply? When we were in the hospital for failure to thrive, it would have been incredibly easy for the doctors to perform "weighted feeds" to calculate how much milk Aubrey was taking in. This would have allowed her to continue nursing even if we still had to supplement with bottles. After we left the practice, I learned the very clear difference between a lactation-friendly vs a lactation-tolerant doctor.

At the end of the day, what it all came down to was this: the people I surrounded myself with were not educated or knowledgeable on how human milk was made or the things that can affect your milk supply. This included: the medical professionals in the NICU, at the pediatrician's office, and in the hospital when we were admitted for failure to thrive.

Is it my family or friends' fault that they didn't know as much as they thought they did on how lactation works? Not at all. This society has not ever set parents up for a successful lactation journey, they were only basing their advice on the advice given to them. And, of course, if you've never had issues with nursing, then how could you possibly know these issues exist? I'll take it even one step further and say that even if issues did arise in previous generations, those parents were just encouraged to formula feed and told they had a low milk supply or their milk wasn't nutritious enough. All the same things I was told with the difference being that I knew better. Something in me always whispered that there was a deeper reason behind the problems we were having. Though Aubrey and I were never able to get back to nursing, I'm glad I never stopped pushing for answers. I will never forgive her first pediatrician for the way she treated us, nor the IBCLC for the lack of support but there was a reason we went through what we did. If not for that incredibly trying journey I would have never written this book.

Sweet Nectar Part II - *Their Stories*

For this second part of Sweet Nectar, I have gathered stories from other parents who have nursed their little one for any period of time from one day to well into toddlerhood. I worked for months searching for stories from all types of parents including BIPOC and Queer parents. I wanted this book to be inclusive with representation to show that chestfeeding does not look the same across the board. This was a safe space for them to tell their stories and be heard without fear of judgement or shame. These stories are written by the parents who lived them and are entirely their own. Welcome to part two *of Sweet Nectar: (Hopefully) Everything You Want to Know About Chestfeeding*.

Baby Blue Eyes

There was no moment more magical than when my son latched onto my nipple the first time, just a few minutes after he was born. I had spent a couple blissful seconds admiring him when I realized… I was in excruciating pain! The feeling was a combination of pinching and pricking. Everyone in the room reassured me that it was normal for breastfeeding to be painful in the beginning, so I continued to feed.

Over the next few hours, every time my son latched, I would gasp in pain. It shocked me how badly it hurt. I had pictured breastfeeding as being a beautiful bonding opportunity, but I found myself dreading his latch every time he was hungry. After our first night in the hospital, my nipples were cracked and bleeding. The nurses offered me a nipple shield, but I found it difficult to use and could tell my son was not getting sufficient milk because of the barrier. I was told to supplement with formula if I felt like he was not getting enough milk through the shield. This meant my only options were painful feeding or supplementation, so I proceeded without the nipple shield.

I was feeling extremely discouraged about breastfeeding only one day into my son's life.

A lactation consultant came into our room on our second day in the hospital and diagnosed my son with a moderate tongue tie by the time he was 24 hours old. I was so grateful toknow that the pain I was experiencing was indeed *not* normal and that there was a solution. However, there was no Ear, Nose, & Throat doctor on call and I was informed I would have to go through my primary care doctor to get a referral. Unfortunately, the earliest appointment we could get was for a week later. That week was full of extremely painful feedings, tearful nights, and much frustration. I went through a lot of nipple butter!

The revision of my son's tongue tie took a total of about 10 seconds at the doctor's office - he didn't cry, and he fed immediately after the appointment. And for the first time - his latch didn't hurt me. I am so proud of myself for never giving up. I never gave into pressure to supplement and I endured hours of painful feedings. I am so grateful to the lactation consultant for diagnosing his tie because if it hadn't been revised, I don't think I would have been able to continue my breastfeeding journey. My exclusively breastfed baby boy is now 2 months old and growing bigger and stronger every day! And now, I can actually enjoy it when I see those baby blue eyes gaze up at me during feedings.

Sofia T.,

United States, She/Her

Body Dysmorphia

I had a home birth, so I have no idea how queer parents, in general, are received by hospital workers. I personally faced many difficulties [including] lip and tongue ties leading to REF and [yeast infections]. [I had] no help at all from professionals. I never met a [professional] capable of helping me. I made it all by myself by searching on the internet and sharing with other moms. That's why I want to become a [lactation] consultant. [I haven't] fully come out yet, so I couldn't see any differences in treatment between me and cis parents, but one thing I felt really hard was body dysmorphia while breastfeeding. Not all the time, but sometimes stronger than others and those times were hell. There [have] been periods of time where all I wanted was to hide my breasts, rip them off [and] never think of them again. My baby was grabbing them all the damn time, playing with my nipples and shit [and] I couldn't say no because he needed them, so all I could do was silently cry. I wanted... needed to wear a binder and again, I could not because I couldn't risk [getting] mastitis. I eventually accepted my body how it is, detached myself from the binary idea that my body is a woman. It is just a body that is mine. I am who I am and I don't care. I don't fit in a binary case and neither does my body, boobs or not.

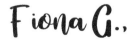

France, Iel (They/Them)

7 Medical Professionals

My son was 14 months old before he got diagnosed with his lip tie. The reason why I thought he had a tie was [because he was] having difficulty breastfeeding and with his latch and [he could only] nurse by using a nipple shield. After my own individual research, the possibility of a lip tie is what seemed to make the most sense to me which is how I came to [address] it to medical professionals. We had 3 pediatricians and 4 lactation consultants miss his lip tie. I was almost certain he had by the time he was 3 months old. After having 7 medical professionals telling me the same thing, I brushed it off as me being a crazy paranoid first time mom and let it go.

Once my son was about 10 months old, I started working in orthodontics and I watched lip ties be diagnosed and it made me think back to my own concerns. Around the same time, my son was cutting his upper teeth and I noticed him having more difficulties cutting teeth than normal, so I decided to look in his mouth again. When looking in his mouth I [saw] something I frequently [saw] at my job. I was almost certain he had a lip tie. I posted a photo on twitter where I had my thoughts confirmed even further. I decided that instead of messing around with more misdiagnoses, I'd take my son to a pediatric dentist. By this time, I was noticing my son was beginning to have issues using straw cups and sippy cups that weren't slow flow as well. My son's speech also had been delayed. After talking to the pediatric dentist they finally gave me the medical diagnosis I had been waiting for. The pediatric dentist also confirmed the lip tie my son had could be causing the issues with sippy cups and his speech. At the point of diagnosis, it felt very bittersweet.

I had worked so hard to try and be heard as a parent to only [be made to feel] crazy. The part that upset me the most was wanting to breastfeed until 1-year-old so badly. My son self-weaned at 6 months old due to his tie. It was upsetting knowing that if the first 7 medical professionals hadn't missed his tie, we would've been able to meet our goal. I was even more upset with myself that I hadn't just taken him to a pediatric dentist in the first place.

The entire experience has been nothing, but a roller coaster of emotions. Once fall comes we're getting his tie cut finally. It's crazy to think that we've been dealing with this for a year and a half now. I'm ready for the whole thing to be over, but I'm glad we finally have answers. The biggest lesson I've learned from this is with all of my children from now on to just go ahead and have them evaluated by a pediatric dentist as soon as possible.

Molly P.,

United States, She/Her

Woman in The Workplace

When I found out I was pregnant, apart from all the other questions, unknown, and excitement, I knew I wanted to breastfeed my child. However, I am not a person who grew up with children in my life, or moms to learn from. So babies and anything related, were like, ahhh! And now, I was going to have one, so anything I learned was really via my own research.

My grandmother raised me, and we never really discussed anything about her pregnancies, or child bearing. The only thing I can remember her telling me, in regards to breastfeeding, is that it helped with her postpartum weight loss, and it helps to shrink the uterus back to size. She always said how it was the most amazing connection to your child you can have, and that my mom was unable to breastfeed because she was an anxious person. So as you can see, my foundation was very weak and confusing. It helped you lose weight, and if you're a "Nervous Nelly" you won't be able to. Awesome.

I read as many books as possible about what to expect with your child, how to calm them when they're upset, sleep training, etc. But I never had any real, valid, resource that truly explained what you would be encountering when breastfeeding. My first real lesson was in the hospital room after my son was born with the lactation consultants. From my readings, I knew to ask the nurses not to bottle feed him when he was born, to let him have skin to skin, and to allow me to breastfeed my child. But as much as you plan, and think you know, everything can change. When I had my son, it was via C-section, which led to complications with me bleeding out. I almost had to have my uterus removed, but luckily it stopped in time to prevent that. Since I was still in the Operating Room and the doctors were figuring out how to stop the bleeding, my baby was taken to the room where they keep newborns and given formula. The nurses, of course, asked me if it was okay to do so, but presented it in a way that I didn't really have an option. It was presented as;

'Well, you can't see your baby for another 3 hours, and he has to eat, so we recommend giving him a bottle, and then we'll help you with breastfeeding once you're able.'

Once I finally was able to meet my little one, I was still recovering from the anesthesia, throwing up, and really out of it. Then coupled with visitors, and family, I felt uneasy about breastfeeding in front of them. Not to mention, I didn't even really know what I was doing. I also didn't realize the first milk that comes out is barely anything, the colostrum was just coming out in droplets, and I felt like I couldn't nourish my child with that. He was born at 9lbs 7oz, and was crying all the time because he was hungry. When I'd ask a nurse for help, they would say oh he has gas, or did you try feeding him and then try to latch him. They didn't explain that it would be so painful, how to correctly latch, or hold him. They didn't explain what to expect, or the process, or if I was doing it right or wrong. They just came in, squeezed my boob flat, pushed his head on to it, and then were like, "okay that looks good, next feeding use the other breast." In my head, I'm like, "Nothing is coming out! What looks good? Is he still hungry, how do I know if he's hungry?" Part of me believes my struggle, in part, had to do with the C-section, because I never truly went into labor. I didn't even dilate. So in my mind, my body didn't receive the typical body cues saying, "Hey, you're about to have a baby, and you're going to need to feed him." The separation after giving birth, I don't think helped either, and his first feeding was via a bottle, I think caused a lot of confusion when I then tried to breastfeed. To say it was stressful and frustrating, is an understatement. I'm not a doctor, nor do I know if my assumption is correct. I'm sure there are many women that have had a C-section that then go on to breastfeed seamlessly. But I just think that naturally, my body wasn't aware of what was going on, and then without the proper support and guidance, I was set up to fail. After realizing my baby was hungry, the nurses convinced me that it was okay to just go ahead and give him a bottle. I'm not going to lie, the relief and also the silence (he stopped crying) from finally being able to feed him a substantial amount, made me think, *'Okay I guess this is what he needs. Who am I to force something that isn't benefiting my child?'* So from there, the lactation consultant noted that I was okay with bottle feeding, and that was the end of any sort of continued instruction in regards to continuing breastfeeding, and what I should expect when heading home. However, I was still inclined to at least try to pump, so that I could give him breast milk, because I had read about the wondrous benefits of breast milk for a baby. So instead of breastfeeding, I would pump enough so that he would have formula for one feeding, and breastmilk for another. My supply wasn't enough to feed him solely with breast milk. I tried a couple more times at home to actually feed him via latching, but he would cry and fight it, and it would end in frustration for both of us, resulting in just going back to the bottle.

I was proud though that I was at least able to give him some breastmilk, so I continued on the journey. I figured as long as he was getting it someway, and was healthy, then what more could I ask for. So I would alternate each feeding between breastmilk and formula. Unfortunately, because my job at the time did not have any initiatives in place to really support maternity leave, or new moms, I had to return to work remotely after two weeks. Having been a workaholic my whole life and not wanting anything to change professionally, before I had my child, I thought this was totally feasible. Boy was I wrong. He was born in September which begins the height of our busy season, so I was completely stressed trying to balance being a new mom, feedings, nap time, and answering the phone and e-mails at the same time. On one particularly stressful day, I couldn't get any milk out when I tried pumping, and at that point my whole supply stopped. I think the lack of knowledge, support, and amount of stress I was under as a new mom attributed to me ending my breastfeeding journey so suddenly. I think it is imperative we create programs and resources for moms that educate the entire process of breastfeeding. It is the most beautiful gift that only we as women are capable of, and yet we are stripped of it, by not being given the knowledge to succeed. I know regardless of how I gave birth, had I been confident enough to tell the nurses, "Hey this is what I want to do and this is how I need to be supported". I think would have started me off in a much better course. As a new mom, you trust the medical professionals and their advice, but deep down I knew that there must've been some better way and I wish I had the confidence to speak up and trust my gut. I hope that any moms reading this who may have had a similar experience, can recognize it's not our fault. We are in a society where breastfeeding is shunned, and we have to personally seek out the resources. But you're not a bad mom if you can't. I had a horrible guilt after my milk supply stopped that I wasn't able to connect to my child enough to continue supplying him food. That maybe I shouldn't have agreed to a C-section and just done it the natural way, or that I didn't research enough. But at the end of the day, as long as your baby is healthy, growing, happy, and nurtured, you're doing a great job. I hope that by reading the resources and educational material and information in this book, you feel supported and confident in your breastfeeding journey. I know that if I have another child, I will surely be relying on this to help guide me through it again.

Greta T.,

United States, She/Her

"Getting Used To It"

Even before I got pregnant, I knew I was going to want to breastfeed my babies. I dreamed about the bond breastfeeding created between mom and baby. Covid-19 really hindered my ability to take classes and prepare for what breastfeeding should look like, andhow to set us up for success. Carter was born a bit early, 36+5, and looking back, I think we attribute some of our earliest struggles to that. We had a smooth, uneventful, medicated (epidural, no induction) vaginal birth, and we had him latched within an hour and a half from birth.

I thought everything was going well, until it wasn't. There was some discomfort as he nursed, but I chalked it up to "my body getting used to it". We saw a lactation consultant in the hospital, and she basically told us his latch was completely wrong and my nipples were bruised because he has basically just been chomping and not truly latching. She worked on some suck training with him, and showed me what a good latch should look like and told us she would come check in with us the next morning to see how things were going. This was just the start of our problems. Overnight, he stopped showing any interest in eating. We were waking him up for each feed, and when he was on the breast, he was very uninterested and it didn't seem like he was getting very much. The nurses were concerned that we had to be waking him for each feed. The following morning, he had his jaundice test, and his bilirubin levels came back high. This gave us some answers as to why he wasn't interested in eating. Basically, when babies are jaundiced, it makes them pretty lethargic and sleepy. I was concerned about my supply because I wasn't pumping much of anything (which I've since learned is zero indication of your supply!), so the nurses suggested I supplement him with formula. I wanted to make sure that he was getting enough into his system, so that he was able to flush the extra bilirubin out. After about 15 hours under the bili lights, we were cleared to go home! Unfortunately, 4 days later at our first pediatrician appointment, they checked his bilirubin levels again and they had spiked, so we were sent back to children's hospital. While there, we were encouraged to strictly breastfeed, so we did! No longer than 3 hours between feeds, and I was only allowed to have him out from under the lights for 30 minutes for each feed. This was super hard because we were still trying to figure out how to latch properly, and it took us quite a few minutes to get what I thought was a good latch, so it was overall pretty stressful trying to nurse him under that time restriction.

Thankfully, 18 hours at children's hospital and we were good as new and sent home (for good this time!). Over the next month or so, we really fought to figure everything out. I was in so much pain, even when using the nipple shield. I didn't know what we were doing wrong, but I knew something was wrong. I was drained. I couldn't handle the pain and the stress of trying to figure this all out tanked my supply. I was SO close to giving up completely. We decided to supplement with formula mix about half and half of formula and my pumped milk, to give my body a break and to give me the opportunity to reset mentally.

At one of his pediatrician follow ups, I told her I was pumping and mixing with formula, because I was having very intense pain if he tried to nurse with their shield and it was unbearable without the shield. I was so frustrated as to why nursing wasn't going well yet. She assessed him for lip and tongue ties and said he had both! I felt so encouraged to hear that, because it meant there was a reason for my discomfort other than us doing something wrong. I also told her I wanted to see an IBCLC, but I couldn't find any doing in person consults. She told me one of their doctors was taking her classes to become an IBCLC, and was in the stage of needing her hours of hands on work with clients to finish out her training. *Finally*! Someone I could see in person to help me out. So, on top of scheduling an appointment with her, we were referred to two different doctors for the tie revisions and we chose who we felt best for our needs. I brought him in for our consultation, and the doctor told us he had a very severe posterior tongue tie, and a minor lip tie that he suspected wouldn't need to be revised. So, we revised his tongue tie that day, and that night I nursed him for the first time with no shield, and no pain. I was so encouraged! I thought we could ditch the shield and that would be the end of it, smooth sailing from here on out. I wish that was the end and it was happily ever after, but not for us. The next day, I was back to being in excruciating pain. I thought the tongue tie reversal was going to be a magical cure all for our issues, and it quickly turned out not to be. Thankfully, we had our visit scheduled with the doctor training in lactation, so I tried not to let it bother me too much. That first appointment was a bust. Baby was so fussy, I'm sure from the revision and just refused to latch while we were there. She told me what to look for in his latch, and sent us on our way since baby wasn't cooperating.

Things still weren't right. We tried to occasionally latch without the shield and it was just an awful amount of pain. It took us another few appointments with that same doctor, but I finally felt like I figured out how to get him latched on right. Slowly, I tried to wean off the shield and once again was met with more pain. I posted in a local breastfeeding group, and they told us to go get checked for thrush. I hate to say it, but I was praying we had thrush. It would have been an answer for the pain and an easy fix. But, no thrush. Basically, our pediatrician said everything looked good and she wasn't sure why I was still having pain, but to try and slowly wean off the shield and come back if it didn't get better. I got in the car after that appointment sobbed. Wasn't breastfeeding supposed to just come naturally? And be easy? Why was it so hard for us? And when the heck was it going to get easier? It felt like never.

Out of desperation, I texted an old friend from high school who I knew is still nursing her two-year-old. I sent her a ridiculous amount of questions and asked her for advice. The simplest thing was about to change my life. Shells. Like the Haakaa brand ones that are meant to collect milk. She said in the beginning, she used those to protect her nipples from the friction of her bra in between feedings and to help keep her nipples dry. I ordered myself a pair ASAP, and it was... LIFE. CHANGING.

The drastic reduction of pain was almost unbelievable. There was still some discomfort as he was still learning how to latch properly now that he has the correct range of motion in his tongue, but the shells made a huge difference. Here we are about 2 weeks after ordering those shells, and we are so close to being completely off the shield! I started very slowly, using it for 95% of the feed, and then taking it off for the last few minutes, and slowly working to have more of the feed without it. His initial latch has the most amount of pain for me, so instead of trying to just grin and bear it, I decided to keep using it at the start of feeds so my nipples didn't get too sore while he still perfected his latch. So, slowly but surely, we went from having the shield on 90% of the time to 75%, 50%, 25%, and now within the last week, we've started working on full feeds without it! It does get to be a lot on my nipples after a while, but overall, it's going really great and I think within the next few weeks I'll be able to fully get rid of the shield!

He's 7 weeks old, and breastfeeding still doesn't fully feel "easy" yet. It's full of learning, struggle, and commitment but it's a commitment I'm so proud to have stuck to. We may not be to the point where fully easy and automatic yet, but we're definitely past the biggest struggles!

Autumn H.,

United States, She/Her

Breastfeeding Chronicles

When I found out I was pregnant with my son, I knew immediately I wanted to breastfeed. I also made sure my husband knew and he was on board. He was so incredibly supportive of the decisions I made while pregnant and during labor/delivery. When I had our son in June of 2019, I had every intention of breastfeeding for as long as possible. In fact, I was looking forward to it. The nurses helped me get my little guy in a feeding position and I thought he was latching. We were moved to my postpartum room where I continued to feed on demand. I thought he was doing great the night he was born. I did request that a lactation consultant come see me in my room to make sure that we were doing things correctly. She showed me some positions and how to hand express.

In the first 24 hours of my son's life, my nipples were so incredibly sore, but everyone told me to keep using the nipple cream and it won't hurt as bad - so I pushed through the pain because I was told it was normal. Within the first week, I started scabbing/bleeding and I DREADED breastfeeding, but I knew it was the best thing for my brand new baby. Although our little guy was gaining weight and growing like anyone would want, I knew in my mama gut he had a lip tie, which was why I had so many issues with pain while feeding. The pediatrician's office dismissed my concerns about a lip tie and told me to keep pushing through after his post-birth appointments. At 13 months old, our pediatric dentist officially confirmed a lip tie. I was so frustrated because I knew if that had been corrected or I was taught how to breastfeed a baby with a lip tie our breastfeeding journey would've lasted until my baby weaned himself.

A couple weeks went by of tears and pain with every feed and then I had a genius idea - I thought that maybe pumping would be a better idea! My son would get the nutrition he needs and I would be able to get some relief. Even then, I just had to wing it and looked things up on Google. Unfortunately, I feel like pumping was even worse, not because it was painful, but I'd pump and within 30 minutes of my session, I was fully engorged and was miserable. I would end up putting baby to breast to help relieve the engorgement and cry through the pain I had from my son's horrible latch. I wanted to reach out to a lactation consultant, but felt like we couldn't afford to have one come to our home. It's safe to say, I felt 100% unprepared when it came to breastfeeding/pumping, it breaks my heart now thinking about it, even 16 months later. I feel like the second baby will have a better chance with breastfeeding since I'm learning so much more about breastfeeding and I also know there is ALWAYS a consultant willing to help a mama in need.

I am so grateful for my amazing husband. He was so supportive and helpful through it all. I can remember crying during breastfeeding sessions because I was hurting so bad. I told him I was considering formula feeding because I was miserable. He never fought me once or questioned my pain, he just asked, "What can I do to HELP YOU?!" Once I made the decision to discontinue breastfeeding, I was heartbroken but relieved at the same time. I loved the connection and bond I shared with my son. I also felt like I was going to receive a lot of hate for not doing something "so natural" but, thankfully, my mom, mother-in-law, and husband supported whatever I felt was best for my mental health and for my baby. My sister, on the other hand, made me feel like I should have tried harder. She was able to breastfeed with no issues and went for quite a while. I know that wasn't her intention, but I couldn't help but feel like a failure when we would speak of our much different breastfeeding journeys.

Lastly, if I could give any advice it would be to reach out and get help- don't feel discouraged if you need help! Breastfeeding should be a happy time with lots of bonding with your new baby. Soak up those moments.

Des S.,

United States, She/Her

Weird Breastfeeding Journey

I had a very strange experience with breastfeeding. When my baby was born, I had her to my breast constantly in the hospital and when she slept, I was pumping. She was getting some at the breast (I knew by her diapers), but I was not able to pump or hand express a single drop of colostrum for 3 days. The pediatrician became concerned she wasn't gaining weight on day 4 and I saw a lactation consultant (LC) on day 5 who inspected baby for ties. She advised me to pump every 2 hours or after each feeding, so I did. All my days were spent nursing baby, then pumping, then bottle feeding colostrum and then going right back to nursing and so on. My milk did not actually come in for five more days. Over those 5 days we had a few weight checks and baby was starting to gain weight very slowly. I am not sure why the doctor never suggested supplementing with formula in those first visits. I feel guilty looking back because my baby was probably hungry.

10 days postpartum, when my milk came in, we did a "weighted feeding," where you weigh the baby before and after nursing to see if they've taken in any milk, and she was taking in milk at the breast. I was relieved, but the LC told me to keep pumping after her feedings to establish a good supply. So, I did that for nearly a month until it seemed like baby was getting full from nursing and no longer wanted a bottle afterwards. After that, I only pumped once a day, getting about 3-4 ounces each time. I'd save that for my husband to give the baby a bottle every day. Breastfeeding was a breeze

until my baby was almost 10 months old and she started only latching in the morning and at night. I would pump 6 times per day for her bottles until a couple weeks later, she would only latch in the morning. Then I pumped 7 times per day, which only lasted a week maximum before I couldn't take it anymore and just started giving her formula and nursing in the morning (while weaning myself off the pump to avoid mastitis). By 10 months old, she was on a full nursing strike and wanted nothing to do with breastfeeding and was exclusively formula fed for 2 months. I had never heard of a baby wanting to quit breastfeeding so young. I have no idea if it was because my supply had dropped or maybe she realized it's easier to get milk from a bottle than the breast and didn't want to put in the effort. It was weird to me, but I did not fight it. Truthfully, I was happy to have my body back to myself.

I am thankful to have been able to mostly exclusively breastfeed my baby, but it was a rough start and I honestly would probably not put myself through that again if I had another baby. I really regret not holding my newborn while she slept instead of pumping constantly. If I could do it over, I'd breastfeed and supplement with formula.

Chloe F.,

United States, She/Her

Finger Feeding Baba

I identify as a white, trans, non-binary, solo parent. I had top surgery by double incision with nipple grafts four years before I gave birth to my kid. I knew it was unlikely I would produce any milk, but it was important to me that my kid get all of the nutrients and benefits of human milk. So, towards the end of my pregnancy, I started collecting frozen milk from multiple generous parents. This was the beginning of what became a full year of driving all over to collect little bags of frozen milk from basement freezers, front door handoffs, and parking lot meetups. I had systems of making sure I defrosted the perfect amount so we never lost a single drop. I am so thankful for the community that helped to feed my kid in the way I chose to.

But the question of how to get that milk to my kid was another issue. My plan was to use a Supplement Nursing System (SNS) at my chest so my baby could latch on to my nipple and be able to suck the milk up through a little tube. I'd spent a long time reading and researching and this seemed like a method many other trans folks had used. However, when the time came, my well researched plan did not seem to work. My grafted nipples are so small and flat that my kid couldn't get a latch at all. I couldn't "squeeze my breast like a sandwich" because I don't have any breasts. I had a lactation specialist come and try to help figure it out. She gave me some nipple shields to use to help get a better latch. But there were just too many moving parts. The nipple shield was impossible to suction to my chest because my chest is flat. If I did manage to get it in place, then I had to hold the tube from the SNS in just the right spot, and then I had to hold my baby in just the right spot and help to get a good latch and I only have so many hands. I was struggling and could not get it to work. I needed a new plan and fast.

I knew bottle feeding was always a potential option, but for me, I wanted that to be a last resort. Because I wasn't giving my baby milk I produced, it felt important to me to have the closeness and connection of feeding from my body. It also felt important to me for my baby to control the flow of the milk and only eat until full. I had researched paced bottle feeding and slow flow nipples, but it was just not the choice I wanted to make for my baby. I had also read that a baby's jaw and tongue development is affected by bottle feeding. Like any parent, I wanted the absolute best for my baby. There were many reasons why bottle feeding was not right for us, but the biggest one was the physical connection I'd be missing.

I had read about a feeding method called finger feeding and decided to give it a try. Essentially, I attached the tube from the SNS to my finger and the baby latched on to my finger and sucked the milk though the tube. It hit all the points I wanted: the baby was in control of the milk flow, it mimicked the sucking motion of being latched to a nipple, and there was a physical connection from my body to my baby. And most importantly, it worked. My baby was eating the proper amount and gaining weight. At first, I thought it was going to be a temporary method until I figured out the nipple shield or some other solution at my chest. I tried several more times over the following days and weeks to get my baby to latch at my chest, but it was always a struggle that ended in a frustrated and hungry baby. And finger feeding just seemed so easy and natural at that point that we stuck with it.

Over the next year, the position my baby was in while finger feeding became a comforting position for both of us, as did sucking on my finger even when there was no tube of milk attached to it. Many nights while falling asleep, my baby would suck on my finger. It was certainly not the feeding plan I had before my baby was born. But it became something that was really special to both of us. One of my favorite pictures of me and my kid from that first year is me sitting on a log in the middle of the woods finger feeding during a backpacking trip. I'm sure there are long term benefits to my kid of choosing to use human milk and choosing to finger feed, but the immediate benefit of having that special physical bond made it worth it for me.

J Carroll.,

United States, They/Them

Community

For my first 2 pregnancies, I was in a heteronormative marriage. I had not explored my own gender and sexual identity. To be fair, I was 23 when I had my first child and was just beginning to understand the working class, white upbringing I had was a bubble. At 8 weeks post C-section with my 2nd child, I found out my husband had not been monogamous. Less than a year later, I found out I was expecting our third while still tandem nursing my two older children. After a nursing discrimination issue in a Dollar General, I was able to tap into a community of nursing folks to support me and I began to realize I had a voice and that agency was possible.

My husband and I were [at] poverty level. It is only, now, looking back years later, I can see the systemic issues affecting my Latinx husband and have been able to let go of a lot of the bitterness I felt over not feeling safe. Realizing if I had had a better language to deal with his mental health issues and crises, things may have been different. At 8 weeks pregnant with my 3rd, we separated and I moved in with my parents. A few months later he was expecting a child with someone else and I felt freedom to finally explore myself. I also felt a deep sense of disconnect from my community, so while I was post op with my 3rd child, recovering in the hospital, I made a promise to myself that I would find a place in our community, Birth Rights Activism and beyond. I loved International Cesarean Awareness Network (ICAN) and the skills I gained in that organization, I felt so hurt and betrayed by the medical establishment in a lot of ways. At the same time, I am so deeply thankful for finding a pediatrician who supported all my choices as I started the solo parenting journey with 3 kids 3 and under. I tandem nursed for almost three years until my oldest was in Kindergarten. I started dating when my youngest was about 6 months. I was lonely, I had met so many wonderful people through taking my children to front line activism events that showed me how different identities could be and be in community together. Through meditations and group circles, I began to trust myself enough to explore who I am. For a time, I was polyamorous, but as my children are still so young, I recognized I do not have the time resources to meaningfully engage in more than one relationship. I explored relationships with partners across the gender spectrum. Some were fascinated that I nursed, some were mortified. I had many conversations in both romantic and platonic relationships about nursing.

Our small family is not perfect, but it is not broken. My youngest just recently weaned at 4 years old. Nursing was a safe place where I could reconnect with my children after going on my own self-love journeys. I miss it, but it feels good to have a firm boundary around my body. Nursing to natural term fostered many conversations with my kids about bodily autonomy and boundaries and I am so thankful I had those opportunities when they were young. It wasn't easy. So many times, I felt like I lost myself in nourishing my kids from my body. I also see now how much of myself I found in the between nursing sessions, how the community

80

that accepted me and my children on our journey is a community that will support us and that we can support as we continue our growth journeys together.

Kris B.,

United States, She/Her

Bodhi's Story

February 2019, my son, Bodhi, was born, making me the one thing I had always wanted to be- a mom. We were thrilled to be a family of three, and so excited for the future. My husband, Aaron, is in the military and we were between bases, staying with my parents at the time of Bodhi's birth. My due date was 2 days before our orders to move from Germany back to the US, so we made the decision that I would leave Germany ahead of my husband to avoid being extended because of the lengthy process of waiting for Social Security cards and infant passports to be able to bring our newborn back to America. We just crossed our fingers that Aaron would make it in time for the birth and thankfully he did. The night Bodhi was born was extremely busy. It was a full moon and according to the labor and delivery staff that meant a lot of babies would be born...they weren't wrong. The lactation consultants on staff were stretched thin. From our very first latch, something was wrong. It was excruciating, my nipples were instantly blistered, bloody, blanched, and flattened into a lipstick shape. We toughed our way through the night until a LC could finally come see us the next day. She came in mid-morning and watched him nurse. "Break the seal, try again. Make sure he is flanging his lip, any time he tucks it under, break the seal, unlatch and try again." That was it. That was all of her advice, and poof she was gone, off to help the next new mom and baby. We were released the next morning, still struggling and trying to flange his lip. Nursing did not get any easier once we were home. My mom's friend has a daughter who is a lactation consultant. She, essentially, had the same advice as the LC in the hospital, and when things didn't improve she finally suggested the use of nipple shields. The shields definitely helped with the pain and blisters I was experiencing, but they were really just a band aid to our problem. Because my parents lived within range of aNavy base, we were forced to take Bodhi there for his well-baby appointments. At his one-week appointment, he still wasn't up to his birth weight, but the doctor wasn't concerned, so neither was I.

Life with our newborn was far from what we imagined. I have spent my life taking care of babies. I started babysitting at the age of 8! I have been a nanny, a lead teacher in a daycare center, and have taken care of more babies and children than I can count and I had never experienced a baby as difficult as my son. He was never happy, he never slept, and he stayed attached to me nursing almost 24/7. When he was around 3 weeks old, my mom suggested we come out to eat with her and a friend. It took over 3 hours just to get out of the house. He just wouldn't stop nursing. He would fall asleep at the breast and then immediately wake up screaming and the whole process would start over again. I remember sobbing to my mom that night and telling her to just go without us. She refused- but it ended up being a really late dinner. By the time he gave up on nursing it was time to put him in his car seat- a whole separate form of torture for both of us. The second he was strapped into a car seat, he screamed bloody murder. I cried the whole torturous way to the restaurant and back home again.

We were making our move from my parents to

our newly purchased home, where my husband was now stationed the day after Bodhi's one-month appointment. The night before his appointment, I developed my first bout of Mastitis. The doctor who saw Bodhi that day and wrote a prescription for antibiotics for me to take and that was that. Bodhi was cleared as healthy and we were free to head to our next base. The trip was hard, Bodhi cried a lot. We had many nursing breaks, and a lot of frustration. But we made it to our new home. Life was just getting harder. My Mastitis kept coming back. We were drowning in spit up. I, basically, lived on the couch with my son attached to my chest. I could not put him down, I could not go to the bathroom without holding and nursing him. I showered almost never, and when I did, I just cried and rushed through because I could hear him screaming on the other side of the wall. A little over a week after we were in our new home, I noticed a pink substance in Bodhi's diaper. My time working with kids told me this was a sign of dehydration. I called the nurse advice line and was told that as long as he was meeting his diaper count, that he was fine, and to just monitor. So that's what we did, he continued to meet the minimum diaper counts and the pink stain went away.

Nine days before Bodhi turned 2 months, I noticed Bodhi's fontanelle suddenly drop. I frantically called the nurse advice line and was instructed to take him to the local emergency room. I called my husband at work, and we rushed to the hospital. Once there they took his weight in kilograms. I didn't think to ask for his weight in pounds, but they should have noticed how poor his weight was for an almost 2-month old who was born at 7lbs 5oz. By the time the ER doctor came in, Bodhi had been constantly nursing for a few hours. The doctor took one look at us and said that he was "nursing perfectly" and to "keep doing what I was doing." He then proceeded to inform us that Bodhi's heart rate was normal, so he was not dehydrated and we were discharged. We didn't know until much later when I went back to ask for his weight that he was, on that day, 7 lbs. 11 oz., just 6 oz. above his birth weight.

On April 19th, we took Bodhi to his two-month well-baby check. When they weighed him he was 7 lbs. 9 oz. The nurse came to ask for a recheck and we got the same weight the second time. I was sobbing before the doctor even came into the room. I had known all along that something was wrong, but was denied over and over again. Bodhi's pediatrician sent us home to pack a bag to head to the big children's hospital in the major city closest to us. He was, technically, admitted for f thrive before we even arrived. I was a wreck, I couldn't help, but to feel like I failed my son. At the hospital, they got me to start pumping. My supply was so low by that point I was only getting about a half ounce combined. So again, I believed it to be my fault. We also began supplementing with formula and between pumping and formula feeding, Bodhi began to gain weight. The on-call LC at the children's hospital was the first person to ever utter the words "tongue tie" to me, and she suspected a posterior tie but was not permitted to diagnose, and the doctors attending to us did not believe there to be ties but knew they didn't really know what they were looking for, so they made an appointment for us to come back and see their Ear, Nose, & Throat Specialist (ENT) once we were released from the hospital for an evaluation. After we were discharged however, the hospital called to inform us that we would need a referral from my son's pediatrician before we could schedule an appointment. Bodhi's pediatrician refused that referral saying that "Tricare only covers anterior ties and she would not put him through the 'trauma' of revision."

The next three months of our lives continued to be a living nightmare. Bodhi was finally gaining weight, but he was still projectile vomiting after every bottle. He genuinely didn't sleep. I could get maybe two 10 minute naps out of him a day, and he had to be laying on me to do so, and he only slept for 30 to 45 minutes at a time at night, and then he would be awake for an hour or two between. It was literal torture. He was almost never happy. The pediatrician just dismissed us saying "most babies grow out of spitting up by 8 months, some babies give up naps early." When Bodhi was almost 5 months old we went home to visit my parents for July 4th. Some other members of my family came as well, including my cousin, a nurse anesthetist, and had her own 5-week-old at the time. She and my aunt witnessed first-hand the struggles we were facing and insisted this was not at all normal and that something was very much wrong. We decided to stop formula at that time and give only breast milk, and that did help some, but it wasn't the real problem. After we arrived home from that visit, I found the Tongue Tied Babies Support Group on Facebook. They saved us. Someone found a provider for us who could perform a functional assessment to determine ties. Bodhi had a posterior tongue tie and an upper lip tie. His ties were finally revised when he was 5.5 months old by the dentist we were referred to from the Orofacial Myologist who diagnosed his ties. We paid out of pocket for the procedure and would do so a million times over. Our lives instantly changed. He began sleeping the same day as his revision. He started taking long naps and sleeping at night. The spit up went almost completely away. He was finally happy. He started smiling and laughing all the time. I had a brand new baby!

I was dumbfounded to learn that his pediatrician is still telling parents that ties are a "fad." She refused to read any of the notes or documents from his assessments or revision. He did need feeding therapy to learn how to properly coordinate his orofacial muscles as he struggled when we tried to start solid, and with feeding therapy I was able to stop pumping and bottle feeding all together and he went back to exclusively nursing at 10 months old- 8 months into exclusively pumping and bottle feeding. He is still nursing like a champ at 22 months old. Body work with a pediatric tie-savvy chiropractor helped to fix his irregular head shape caused by the ties, remove the leftover tension in his body so he could finally ride comfortably in a car seat, and she was able to help flatten his pallet. When our next child is born, we are going to go straight from the hospital to the incredible team that saved us. Never again will we suffer like we did with Bodhi. I feel so guilty that his first almost 6 months of life were such a painful existence. Our children are beyond resilient, but no baby should be forced to suffer over something so fixable.

Kylie W.,

United States, She/Her

Mission "Impossible"

Breastfeeding was important to me. This seems unusual in transgender men. Most seem to tolerate breastfeeding at best, willing to endure it to provide for their child, but I wanted it badly. Not just for my child, but for myself. Part of this was interwoven with my regret for my top surgery. What came first, my regret from my surgery, or my disappointment at being unable to feed my baby? It's hard to tell sometimes, but they certainly influenced each other. I hated that I wouldn't be able to breastfeed "right". Even ten months on, as I've discovered alternatives to almost every part of breastfeeding, it still feels incomplete.

Three years before getting pregnant, I had double incision with nipple grafts—not only was the tissue of my breasts removed, the nipples were removed and reattached, making breastfeeding, according to multiple surgeons and lactation consultants and transgender people, impossible. After stopping testosterone, I had little optimism for being able to breastfeed. But once my period returned, I found that around ovulation, there would regularly be a small discharge from my nipples. That gave me some hope. I also felt hope after talking with a lactation consultant who was very involved with the transgender community. She acknowledged she didn't have the answers, but she put in a lot of research to help me.

She had hope, and so I did, and she easily told me I had options, and if it ended up not happening, it was fine.

I knew that intellectually, but I still wanted it. I needed it to feel better about my body. That seems selfish sometimes, like I put my own priorities above my child's, even in this. But I'm at a point, now, where I can acknowledge those feelings, and acknowledge my own healing is just as important as my baby's needs, especially when they coincide so smoothly. During my pregnancy, I heard a lot about breastfeeding. I was on WIC, and they pushed it so hard. I cried after our meeting, because they didn't seem to realize that that wasn't going to happen for me, and it hurt to hear about it. I felt like I was setting myself up for failure. When reading pregnancy books, I skipped chapters on breastfeeding, knowing it would be painful, then returned to read them because I wanted to know, I wanted to pretend, I wanted to hope. As my due date neared, I talked to my hospital. I was worried that they would refuse to let me breastfeed, since I had so little chance of success, and even that success would certainly be mediocre at best. They were very open to letting me breastfeed. Just in case, though, knowing how important this was going to be to me, I got a note from my Lactation Consultant talking about our plans to do combination feeding, with the primary focus being skin-to-skin.

My child's birth was challenging and traumatic, but the best moment was when I held him in my arms after the emergency C-section. I held my breast in my hand—while 'flat', I still had a decent amount of tissue left behind, one of the reasons my lactation consultant was optimistic. I was stunned when my child immediately latched without a problem. It was his first gift to me. My body responded by giving me another gift, as the pediatrician commented that he was getting colostrum right away. That beautiful first moment of perfection later spiraled. The hospital ignored all my wishes to breastfeed. They ignored the note from the lactation consultant (who did have experience with my situation, while they did not) and never contacted her. They acted like I was starving my child, even though I was combination feeding from the beginning, which only made my complex feelings around my chest more so.

The hospital sent in another lactation consultant who insisted on pumping to the point that she took my child from my arms and so I could pump. (Yup, you read that right.) I had a C section, and putting my child right next to me might as well have been taking him from the room for the effort it would take to retrieve him. She did this even though I stated pumping was not working and the main goal was skin-to-skin, even though they themselves said I would not be successful. Any time I tried to breastfeed, someone was there making it difficult and telling me to stop. They later sent me home with instructions that my doctor—who saw me through my transition and is my child's pediatrician and a family doctor—called a load of crap and immediately threw away, a sentiment I fully supported and appreciated.

I was relieved to return home so I could resume this very important goal of mine. Instead, my child now refused to latch. I can't say for sure, but to this day, I insist the issues at the hospital contributed to this sudden change in his attitude towards breastfeeding. At least I continued to lactate. I was dissuaded at first, after my time at the hospital, but my chest was visibly swollen and aching, so I decided to try again. This ended up not working, and was so stressful for both my child and I that I gave it up. I was too depressed, with complicated feelings about "my failure" and likely some postpartum stress, to contact my lactation consultant. I did manage to salvage my experience, though, hand expressing drops at a time and finger feeding them to my child. I had heard even a drop helped, so I did this diligently for several weeks. I wish I had done it longer, wish I had tried harder, though I do believe I made the right choice for both of us at the time. At that point, I started searching for donor milk. The hospital had dissuaded me from this, which my lactation consultant later was shocked by and believes was discrimination. I didn't have high hopes of finding donor milk, since I don't drive, but I was able to exclusively feed him this way for six of my child's first eight months. I don't even know how I managed other than through determination and help, but I am grateful for this. Each donor bottle was a mix of emotions—triumph for obtaining this liquid gold, and failure for not providing it myself.

I had a birth reclaiming ceremony a couple months ago. During it, I spoke with my doula and the doula leading the ceremony about all the disappointments involved with my child's birth. But I also acknowledged the positives. One of the biggest for both of these was feeding my child. I was so disappointed and depressed that I wasn't able to feed him "properly," that I could've, but made a choice three years ago that resulted in me not being able to, a choice I regret.

However, my body has shown itself to be incredible. To this day, any time I tell people that I was able to feed my child anything (and still lactate a little around ovulation), they are disbelieving. They say it's impossible. Well, then my body is impossible, because it succeeded.I did something I shouldn't have been able to do. *I love my body for that.*

Ryden A.,

United States, He/Him

Dysphoric Milk Ejection Reflex

My breastfeeding journey started out normal with little to no issues. I remember the lactation specialist came into my Hospital Room and then didn't stay very long at all. I had been researching my whole pregnancy and maybe it was my fault for not asking more questions, but she watched me feed my son for what felt like only 5 minutes and told me he had a good latch and left. We never saw her again. When we got home is when my son started to nurse longer. I knew all about cluster feeding so [I] was prepared for this and would latch him and use my Haakaa on the other side and it was all good. This is the time period (the 1st few nights at home), I noticed an increase in my anxiety while feeding him. I would get extremely agitated and feel uncomfortable even though our latch was fine. My partner would bring me water as I would also feel super dehydrated, and eventually it would subside. As I got more comfortable on my breastfeeding journey, I started to double pump while my son slept after feeds and that is when I noticed an increase even more so in the "anxiety" as I would come to understand it. This is the hardest part to explain, as everything was going so smoothly and I had such [an] amazing newborn I would feel so completely agitated and feel aggression toward my partner while I pumped. I'd feed my son and my anxiety would kick back in times 10 and it wasn't just anxiety this time it was different. I'd go from rage to tears and felt very not in control. I thought I had prepared for every obstacle possible that could hit our breastfeeding journey, but I was wrong and I was fully ready to stop breastfeeding because of the emotions and how they started to consume me.

At that point in time, I was pumping after every feed or while my son was napping. I would never even feel fully empty and I would always just end up ending my session exactly after 20 to 25 minutes. After speaking to not 1 but 3 lactation specialists through WIC and my doctor, we realized I was hitting my 2nd letdown and those emotions would kick in around that time. [At] I was also in therapy, as well, 1 to 2 times a week and we had been talking about supplementing and trying meds. I felt like I was failing on my breastfeeding journey and back to wanting to give up. After a lot of talk and a few more weeks of trial and error, supplementing formula was sadly unsuccessful and I was told to try and just continue our breastfeeding journey and cut all the extra pump sessions and see how that went. After 2 weeks of that, things truly started to get better mentally for me. Now when I feed my son I experience 30 seconds to 2 minutes max of emotional discomfort and am able to use coping skills I learned in DBT and therapy to push forward and realize it will pass.

I've been sober for 2 years and 5 months and this journey was by far one of the hardest journeys I've ever been on. I am so grateful for all the lactation specialists and doctors who were on my side in continuing this breastfeeding journey and with all the support we were able to overcome those bumps and my son is now thriving 21 pounds and exclusively breastfed.

Katie Z.,

United States, She/Her

Exclusively Pumping

When we finally conceived Clementine, my pregnancy was so easy. We'd been trying for almost a year, with five failed Intrauterine Insemination (IUI), one failed in-vitro fertilization (IVF), switched donors and got lucky on our second IVF (with the original donor)! My wife and I were elated. We made every appointment, did all of the testing and screening, so we're totally unprepared when our daughter was born with a surprise cleft in her soft palate. Throughout my entire pregnancy, I'd been looking forward to having that amazing breastfeeding and bonding relationship I'd read so much about. Clementine's type of cleft made it impossible for her to nurse. The first few days after she was born were a whirlwind as Clementine went into the special care nursery for extra monitoring to rule out other potential issues. During that time, I began pumping regularly.

I was completely unprepared for what to expect as I embarked on what would be a 10.5-month journey of exclusive pumping. We were fortunate that she did not need feeding tubes, but she did require a special feeder nipple and careful feeding to ensure that milk did not goup the hole in the back of her mouth and up out her nose. There was a learning curve for all of us.

Exclusive Pumping (EP) was a long and lonely journey for me. Although I had 100% support from my wife, I felt sad and disappointed and an enormous, and unhealthy, weight to do everything I could to feed only breastmilk even if it meant pumping every two hours around the clock and what seemed like endlessly washing bottle and pump parts just in time to start the process all over again. I felt so much societal pressure with all of the "breast is best" messaging I'd seen that formula equaled failure in my mind. This is a load of garbage; you are not a failure if you formula feed your baby. We did supplement and eventually turned to formula when I couldn't take pumping any longer and I don't regret it one bit.

Pumping took a toll on my body, as well as, my mind. Being new parents, we were struggling to figure out our new routines. Like many before us, remembering to brush our teeth in the morning was a major feat. I was so focused on feeding the baby, I regularly forgot to feed myself. I struggled the entire time I pumped. Looking back, I should have gone to talk to someone about postpartum depression, but I was too afraid to admit it. I felt all alone and none of the mom friends I had and mom groups on Facebook were of any help. Online, I was made to feel like feeding my baby pumped milk was not breastfeeding and that it wasn't possible to really bond without the baby to boob physical connection. I guess I bought into that as I still somewhat am grieving not being able to nurse my first baby. I found some solace and community when I discovered a EP Facebook group. These were other mothers who were experiencing the same issues and sometimes heartache as I was. It was a support group for only other "EPers" like me that I wasn't able to find anywhere else.

Community is important even if it comes in the form of total strangers. Regardless of how supportive my wife and friends and family were, I needed to be able to share and ask questions of others traveling a path similar to mine.

What hit me hardest was how I felt more connected to my pump then I did to my baby. In the end I exclusively pumped for 10.5 months. I was hooked up to the machine for 574 hours (almost 24 whole days), pumped a total of 15,824 ounces (almost 124 gallons) and donated 1,800 ounces. I pumped at home all hours of the day. I pumped in the car to and from work daily. I pumped at work, in airports, on airplanes, on car trips, at family parties, friend's houses, at doctor's offices, in parking lots, and many other places I can't remember at this moment. When we started talking about having a second child, I decided that if they couldn't nurse, I wouldn't EP again and would formula feed instead.

When looking back on Clementine's first year and thinking about exclusive pumping... Was it worth it? Absolutely. Would I do it again? No way!

Gwendolyn H.,

United States, She/Her

Sweet Nectar Part III

I thought long and hard about what I wanted to include in this book. After becoming aware of all of the misinformation about chestfeeding on the market, it became increasingly more important for me to use the knowledge I have gained through my schooling to help educate a wider audience. The next 45 pages will go into the many misconceptions of the human milk supply and nursing, as well as, tips and tricks to help you have the best experience nourishing your child with your milk. I hope that you find this section easy to read and the information easy to retain. Welcome to part three *of Sweet Nectar: (Hopefully) Everything You Want to Know About Chestfeeding.*

Getting Prepared

I am a firm believer in doing as much preparation as possible before setting out on any journey and chestfeeding is no exception. It's so important to be prepared for anything that may arise. So many parents don't do research or take a class until they are faced with an obstacle but why wait until then? This section will cover the many ways you can prepare yourself for a positive chestfeeding journey!

Finding Your Care Team

Finding the right hospital to deliver at and the right doctor to care for your child is so much more overwhelming than I think any new parent is prepared for. Do you deliver at the same hospital that your mother-in-law did? Or, do you choose the pediatrician who has been in your family for years? There are so many options that making a choice feels impossible. Luckily, there are a few things that, when kept in mind, can help to make the process a little easier.

There is a wonderful movement called the "Baby-Friendly Hospital Initiative" (BFHI) that was founded by the World Health Organization (WHO) and the United Nations Children's Fund (UNICEF) in 1993. This initiative was set into motion with the goal of creating a labor and delivery environment that benefited both birthing person and baby in the best way possible by optimizing their chestfeeding experience. In other words, they want to make sure every birthing person who delivers at a Baby-Friendly hospital is set up for success! Before this initiative, it was very common for hospitals to take the baby to the nursery after being delivered, give each parent a package with formula samples before they left and encourage the use of bottles. The BFHI has established guidelines for these Baby-Friendly hospitals to follow such as allowing baby to room-in with their parent, restricting the free formula offered, providing parents with chestfeeding [information] and so much more. The website: **babyfriendlyusa.org** has all of the information on what it truly means to be a Baby-Friendly hospital and how to find one!

Well, there's half the battle right? You know where to look for a hospital that will support you on your journey but what about a pediatrician? As made clear in both parts I and II of this book, pediatricians are often not knowledgeable on chestfeeding or how to handle a problem when faced with one. So that leaves the question: How do I know my child's pediatrician will be supportive? This answer isn't as straightforward as finding a Baby-Friendly hospital to deliver, but that doesn't mean there isn't an answer! When looking for a pediatrician who will support your chestfeeding journey you can ask some of the following questions --

Does this office have a lactation consultant available that this office refers parents to?

Having a lactation consultant in the office or building means this is an office that values the opinion and guidance of one. Sometimes offices aren't large enough to accommodate a lactation consultant though, so having one they regularly work with and refer to is the next best thing.

Does this office use the WHO growth chart or the Center for Disease Control (CDC) growth chart?

This question is important; I can't stress it enough. When doctors document your child's growth there are two charts they may use. One was created by the WHO and the other was created by the CDC. Unlike the chart from the CDC, the chart created by the WHO is based on how a baby who is nourished by human milk grows, which is very different from how a baby who is nourished by formula grows. You want a pediatrician who uses the WHO chart because that means they acknowledge that using human milk should be the standard for feeding your baby and will not expect them to be growing like a formula fed baby does.

By simply asking those two questions, you will have a better idea of if the pediatrician you want to choose for your child is chestfeeding friendly.

Writing Your Birthing Plan

One of the most important things you can do to not only prepare yourself for chestfeeding, but labor and delivery is creating a birthing plan. This is a document that you give to your doctor or midwife before you deliver and sometimes the nursing staff will ask you for a copy on the day you go into labor. You can include requests like: what position you want to deliver in, how many people and who is allowed in your room, your preference for pain management and more. It's relatively simple to google different templates for a birthing plan and then add what you want or take out what you don't want but what I want to focus on is how you can set yourself up for chestfeeding success with one.

You'll probably notice that in many of the templates you find online, birthing plans are usually separated by sections like "Labor" "Delivery" and "Postpartum." If you cannot find a birthing plan with a section for how the baby should be fed I highly suggest adding one in. Here are the main things you want to be sure to include:

I would like to allow my baby to do the 'breast crawl' after delivery.

Our babies are capable of more than most parents realize. When given the opportunity newborns do what is called the "breast crawl" within the first 90 minutes following their birth. They use all of their senses to find your chest and latch on to your nipple. The scent that the oil glands on your nipples give off allow your baby to smell where they are going. The new, larger size of your areola serves as a sort of "bulls eye" visual for them to track down with their eyes. The sound of your heartbeat is a familiar one they instinctively follow. All of this allows your baby to slowly, but surely make their way up your body to latch on to your chest for the first time!

This is an incredible moment that, when allowed, gives your baby a very positive first experience with nursingand will help with confidence in nursing for both of you down the road!

I would like to delay any vaccination, baths or measurement taking until after the first nursing session.

Delaying these routine procedures allow for birthing person and baby to really have a moment to themselves, uninterrupted. The first nursing session within those 90 minutes is so essential for establishing a full milk supply.

* Please send in a lactation specialist immediately after birth.

This one is, especially, helpful if you don't have a midwife or doula or if you do, but they do not have any sort of lactation training. A lactation consultant in the hospital will help remind you of how to latch your baby, as well as, different positions you may want to try. I put as asterick by this one because even if you put it in your birthing plans, sometimes hospitals get very busy and you may need to remind the nurses of your request.

Please do not give my baby a pacifier.

Now, each lactation consultant will have a different opinion on pacifiers for chestfeeding babies. I am a firm believer in waiting until a chestfeeding relationship is well established (usually after 6 weeks) before introducing any sort of artificial nipple to a baby for a few reasons. Pacifiers can cause nipple confusion in some babies and, therefore, make it difficult for them to stay interested in latching. Additionally, pacifiers can make you miss early hunger cues such as baby sucking on their fingers or smacking their lips. Until you become very familiar with your baby's hunger cues, I suggest limiting pacifier use.

If my baby should end up in NICU please use alternative feeding methods such as a cup, spoon or syringe before using a bottle.

This is another great way to help reduce the odds of nipple confusion or preference. Until a chestfeeding relationship is well established, I highly suggest alternative feeding methods whenever possible. If you are delivering at a Baby-Friendly hospital, this should be no problem! If you are not, the most important thing you can do is advocate for yourself. Make sure you know how to do these alternative feeding methods yourself so that you can show the hospital staff.

Remember, they work for you!

If alternative feeding methods are not available, please make sure that my baby is pace-fed with a bottle on a slow flow nipple.

Sometimes, alternative feeding methods are just not available because the hospital might not have the necessary equipment. When this happens, don't panic! There is another way that you can help prevent nipple confusion and it's called "Paced-Feeding". We'll go more into exactly what it is and how to do it in another section.

If my baby has to be taken to the NICU please have a pump waiting for me in recovery so that I can pump as soon as I am able.

As I briefly mentioned above, allowing your baby to latch and nursing within those first 90 minutes after birth are so important for bringing in a full milk supply. However, that isn't always an option, especially for birthing people whoose babies have to be taken to the NICU. The next best thing is requesting for a pump to be waiting for you in recovery so you can pump as soon as you are able to and start getting colostrum and milk to your baby!

The most important thing to take away from this section is to be your own advocate. Hiring a doula to help with your labor and delivery can really take the pressure off of having to remember all of these things yourself. But, even though a lot of states have free doula/birthing companion programs, not all do and it may not always be affordable for a birthing person to hire one. Having a well thought out and easy to read birthing plan that outlines your plans for feeding your infant makes it easy to have your requests voiced and concerns heard.

Chestfeeding Expectations

So, we've talked about how to prepare yourself for your journey, but what exactly can you expect? There are so many things that I wish had been explained to me prior to delivering my baby. I had a lot of expectations for what pumping would look like, how long it would take my milk to come in... The list goes on. In this section, we will cover most of those expectations so you can be prepared for what chestfeeding will most likely look like immediately and in the first few weeks after delivery.

Leaking

Starting from 16 weeks' gestation, your body is ready to produce a full milk supply, so it's no surprise that around this time a lot of parents experience some leaking. This is completely normal and may continue throughout your entire chestfeeding journey or it may stop at any point. I really want to make it clear though that just because you used to leak and at some point the leaking stopped does not mean that you are losing your milk supply. In fact, some parents never leak and that is completely normal too!

If you start to notice leaking any earlier than 37 weeks do not pump or try to squeeze it out! This is very important to remember. Nipple stimulation is a great way to naturally induce labor and you wouldn't want to do that prior to making it to full-term (37 weeks).

Though leaking can happen at any point past 16 weeks (sometimes earlier for a second or subsequent pregnancy) it's much more common to happen after a full milk supply is established. There are a lot of things that can cause leaking, but the most common causes are engorgement, nipple stimulation and hearing your baby (or sometimes any baby) cry. Don't be surprised if you find yourself leaking after hearing another baby cry at the grocery store!

There are so many choices for chest pads to use so that you don't leak through your shirt. From disposable to washable, all you have to do is pick which style works best for you!

How Milk Supply Works

I wanted to make this section one of the first because I strongly believe this is the most important information for a new parent who plans on chestfeeding.

For the first 6 weeks (give or take) your postpartum hormones are what are primarily responsible for milk production. Oftentimes this means that you may have a bit of an oversupply to start off. After those first 6 or so weeks, your milk supply will primarily be dependent on supply and demand. This means the more you latch your baby or pump the more milk you will produce. There are other factors that affect your milk supply, as well, like water and caloric intake, but we'll go into more detail about those a bit later.

As a general rule of thumb, you can expect to notice that the more you remove milk from your chest the more milk you will produce.

Milk Production Supplements

Oftentimes one of the first things a new parent wants to invest money in is supplements to help maintain or increase milk supply. There is an entire industry that preys off of parents who don't know any better. From teas to brownies, cookies and shakes, there is a wide assortment of supplements to choose from.

How do you know which is the right one for you?

The short answer is, *none of them are.*

The only thing that is 100% proven to increase your milk supply is "supply and demand" just like I mentioned in the section above. Now, does this mean that there has never been a parent to benefit from these supplements? Not necessarily. The placebo effect is a very powerful thing so it's not surprising that some parents have seen positive results after consuming these supplements. However, the reverse is also true. There are very common ingredients in a lot of the supplements in stores today that have actually beenproven to cause a decrease in milk production.

Indulging in a "lactation cookie" or special drink may seem harmless, but when there's no proof how much "good" it can do, why risk the chance of any damage being done?

Onset of Milk Production After Delivery

For some reason there is this crazy misconception that you will have a full milk supply immediately after delivering your baby. While it's true that your body is ready to produce a milk supply starting at 16 weeks pregnant, and you may even begin to start leaking, it takes a few days after delivery for your mature milk to come in. On average, for a vaginal delivery it takes an average of 3-5 days for your mature milk to come in. If you have a c-section delivery it can take up to 10 days, but on average you can expect your mature milk to be in 5-7 days after delivery. Now I know what you're thinking: "How does my baby eat while I'm waiting for my mature milk?" That's a valid question and luckily, the answer is not "formula."

Before your mature milk comes in you will produce something called *colostrum*. This nutrient and antibody dense liquid is a darker, almost golden yellow color compared to the off white of your mature milk. It's also thicker, meaning a little goes a long way! In the first few days of life a baby needs far less milk than you may think and colostrum is the perfect "cocktail" of nutrients to nourish your baby until that mature milk comes in. Over the course of the days leading up to your full supply coming in, you may begin to notice the milk changing color if you're pumping! You may also notice the color of your baby's stool changing to eventually land on a yellow, mustardy color with little seeds. This stool is consistent in babies fed with mature human milk!

Engorgement After Delivery

It is completely normal to experience a degree of chest engorgement around the same time your milk comes in. It may be uncomfortable, but it should never be unbearably painful. The best thing to do when this happens is latch your baby or pump as much as possible to relieve the engorgement. It's important to remember, though, that you only need to do one or the other. There is no need to pump, if you are regularly latching your baby. Now there are some instances where a parent's baby might be in the NICU and they only latch for a few sessions a day, in which case pumping is necessary to

110

make up for those lost sessions and maintain a milk supply.

If you're still not finding relief with just latching/pumping, a warm compress can be used before a session to help with discomfort and a cold compress and be used afterwards. Warm showers are your best friend and hand expressing between sections is always extremely beneficial.

"My Chest Doesn't Feel Full Anymore. Am I Losing My Milk?"

Remember when I mentioned a few sections back that for the first 6 or so weeks your milk supply is mostly dependent on your postpartum hormones? Well, because of this and the temporary oversupply that often comes with it, parents sometimes notice around that time that their chest doesn't feel as full between feedings anymore. This may cause a moment of doubt or the feeling that your milk supply is dropping but that couldn't be further from the truth! At this point, your milk supply has adjusted to exactly what your baby needs based on how they've been nursing (or you've been pumping) since the delivery!

There's a saying in the lactation world that goes, "A soft chest is a working chest." There's a huge myth that if your chest isn't full and engorged all the time that means you aren't making enough milk when in reality, it's quite the opposite. When your chest is full of milk, leaving you with that full or engorged feeling, your body sends a message to your brain telling it to stop making milk. Meaning, when your chest is soft, your brain is telling your body to keep making milk! Isn't it amazing how that works? So, try not to panic when you make it to that 6-week mark and your chest feels softer than you're used to, all it means is that your body is doing exactly what it's supposed to be doing.

Delivery & Hospital Stay

By now, I hope you have started to develop a basic understanding of how lactation works and what to expect in those early weeks. In this section, we'll touch on what your experience may look like after delivery and while you're still in the hospital.

Golden Hour

Okay, so the name here might be a little misleading but "Golden Hour" refers to that first 90 minutes after your baby is born. This is when something called the "Breast Crawl" takes place where your baby will quite literally crawl to your chest. After they reach your chest there is a very specific sequence of events that takes place during this crucial time, let's break it down.

6 minutes after contact- baby opens their eyes

11 minutes after contact- baby begins to massage the chest

12 minutes after contact- baby begins hand & mouth play (sucking on hands and fingers)

21 minutes after contact- baby beings rooting (lookingside to side)

27 minutes after contact- baby's tongue will begin to stretch to lick your nipple. This phase is the longest!

80-90 minutes after contact- your baby has latched and is now nursing!

After this first nursing session, your baby will likely fall asleep for 2-5 hours. This is known as the "Recovery Sleep". You've both been through a lot so if you can, try to sleep during this time too! If this is your first baby, it might be hard but try to resist staying awake to watch your little one sleep. You'll have plenty of time to do that at home!

Now don't worry if you have a c-section, the "Breast Crawl" is something that can be done after you feel well and alert enough to hold your baby.

Latching After Golden Hour

Now that first latch is often blissful. The moment you were dreaming about your entire pregnancy has finally come! But what if it's not? What if you feel intense nipple pain when your baby latches on? Well, this can indicate a problem. Like I mentioned in an earlier section, having a lactation consultant sent to your room immediately after delivery is extremely beneficial. In this instant, a lactation consultant should be able to assess what is causing the pain. Remember, chestfeeding should *never* hurt. Sure, it may be an uncomfortable or odd sensation that you aren't used to, but if it hurts, there is a problem. Whether it's the way the baby is latched or positioned, or something more technical like a higher than normal palate or an oral tie of some sort. Make sure you mention this to the lactation consultant as soon as you notice it!

Skin-To-Skin

Skin-to-skin is such a crucial part of feeding your

baby with your milk, whether you are nursing or pumping! It not only has benefits for your baby, but for you as well. Skin-to-skin contact has been proven to lower stress hormones in baby and parent, promote bonding, stabilize infant heart rate and temperature, and even maintain your milk supply!

You can do skin-to-skin anytime you feel like bonding with your baby, but it's especially beneficial right before a nursing or pumping session to help promote a milk let down. It's also been found that placing a baby on your chest while they are upset can help to settle them! Just make sure both you and the baby are covered with a blanket or two, you don't want to get cold!

Postpartum Contractions

Yes, you read that right. There is such a thing as contractions after you've given birth. Your uterus doesn't deflate like a balloon immediately after delivery so in order for it to shrink back to a "normal" size, it contracts similar to how it does when you're in labor. Now of the many benefits of nursing, one of them is actually these contractions. Remember when I mentioned that nipple stimulation can trigger you to go into labor? That's because nipple stimulation causes contractions! These contractions that happen while you're nursing after delivery are what help your uterus to shrink back down! They aren't as painful as labor contractions but that doesn't mean they're pleasant. Something that I always found helpful was making sure that my bladder was completely empty before I pumped or latched my baby on. Don't worry, these contractions don't last for long and should stop before your mature milk even comes in!

Hands-Free Nursing

Swaddling has become such a regular practice for most American families. It's thought to mimic the snugness that your baby felt in the womb and help them transition to the world easier. Some parents even think it helps their baby sleep longer, but there is a crucial point often not mentioned when it comes swaddling while nursing. Babies use their hands to nurse! We've gotten so used to swatting their hands away, holding them back, putting mittens on them or even going so far as to swaddling baby while they nurse, but all of these things can actually make it harder for your baby to nurse! Think about it this way, when you're drinking a milkshake you have to use your hands right? You hold the cup, maybe even the straw and sometimes you might swirl the milkshake around in the cup to loosen it up and make it easier to drink. This is sort of how you baby will use their hands to help them nurse. At first, it may look a little disorganized and erratic but over time, with practice, they learn to control their hands and use them to massage your chest which helps to stimulate your milk glands and produce more milk!

So when your mother-in-law or cousin's best friend tells you that it's better to swaddle your baby while they nurse, you can tell them what you know. The more your chest is stimulated while nursing or pumping the more milk you will release and produce. This can only happen when your baby's hands are free from restriction. Allowing your baby to nurse hands free lets them practice what they're born to do!

How Will I Know When My Baby Is Hungry?

What a common question for new parents. Babies cry for all sorts of reasons so how do you know when they're crying because they're hungry? This answer might surprise you but if they're crying because they're hungry then that means you've missed every other sign. Crying is a late hunger cue, meaning it only happens after your baby has tried every other way of telling you they're hungry. Here are all the ways your baby will tell you they are hungry well before theystart crying:

Stirring- If your baby seems relatively calm one moment and the next you notice restless movement, this can be considered "stirring."

Mouth Opening/Smacking lips- Sometimes babies makea face that resembles a fish opening and closing their mouth. As silly and cute as this looks, it's actually your baby saying, "Hey! I'd like some milk please!"

Rooting- I mentioned rooting briefly in the section on "Golden Hour". When a baby is rooting, that means they are moving their head side to side searching for something (your chest or a bottle) to latch on to.

Sucking on Fingers/Hands- This tends to be the last early hunger cue before your baby starts to cry. By this point, they are sucking on anything that is close to their face, which is typically their fingers and hands.

Now, as your baby grows past the newborn stage, some of these early cues may start to fade or mean something other than, "I'm hungry," but typically by that point you'll have gotten to know your baby well enough to be able to tell when sucking on their fingers is a hunger cue or just self-soothing. Following these early hunger cues in the first few weeks of life is crucial for developing trust with your baby and making sure that your milk supply stays consistent in meeting your baby's demands!

Cluster-Feeding & Comfort Nursing

Cluster-feeding is when a baby feeds for longer than normal sessions, or more frequently, than normal. It can start as early as before your mature milk even comes in, which is why I included it in this section. Even though it is very common for nursing babies, it can cause parents to feel like they are losing their milk. Rest assured, this is a normal part of development! It may happen a few times over the course of your chestfeeding journey. This is just your baby's way of telling your body to make a little extra milk than its use to making. In the early days, before your mature milk comes in, this is what helps to bring it in! The most common reasons for a baby to cluster-feed include: growth spurts, developmental leaps, illness and comfort! Remember, your baby is not using you as a "pacifier" a pacifier is made to mimic the human nipple.

I'm Home! What Now?

So, now you're home and everything is different. No more nurses or doctors checking on you every few hours, but that also means you don't have their guidance anymore. Understandably, a lot of new parents are nervous to go home and, even more so, when they are chestfeeding.

Is My Baby Getting Enough Milk?

One of the biggest concerns chestfeeding parents have is whether or not their baby is getting enough milk. If you aren't pumping to give your baby bottles it can be difficult to gauge how much milk they are taking in. It's important to remember that what goes in must come out! The only way to tell how much milk your baby is taking in is by how much comes out.

During the first seven days of life, your baby may only have 1 wet diaper for every day that they've been alive. So this means on day two they'll have two wet diapers, on day four they'll have four and so on.

Four tablespoons is what a "full" wet diaper is considered to be, which can look different depending on the size of the diaper. If you're unsure, simply measure out 4 tablespoons of water and pour it into a diaper so you can feel about how heavy it is. After the first week your baby should have about 8-12 wet diapers a day. Again, this will vary depending on how much the diaper holds and how often you change it. Additionally, your baby should be having about one diaper with stool every few days. It's normal to have several a day for the first few weeks, but eventually, babies fed human milk can go up to a whole week without having a bowel movement! Keep that in mind, but check with your doctor if you think your baby is constipated.

In addition to monitoring your baby's diaper count, you can also be sure they are getting enough milk by asking their pediatrician for their growth chart.

Every baby will be somewhere different on the chart, but what's most important is that they are staying on the same growth curve. Fluctuating up and down a little bit is normal, but, generally speaking, if your baby is in the 71st percentile after you leave the hospital and then at the two-month checkup they are in the 30th percentile then that is a red flag. Talk to your doctor about the best way to supplement until your baby is back on their growth curve.

How Long Should My Baby Nurse On One Side?

Sometimes hospitals have a new parent keep track of how long a baby is latched on to their parent or you might have even heard from a family member "don't let them nurse for more than 10 minutes on one side." There's a belief that if your milk supply will be uneven or your baby might not get enough milk if they only nurse on one side. How much truth is there to this? Well, not much at all. The human body does an amazing job at regulating your milk supply to exactly what your baby needs! There is never any need to limit the amount of time they spend latched to one side. You should always allow your baby to fully finish nursing on one side. Don't unlatch them, but let them unlatch themselves. You can absolutely offer the other side, but if they don't take it respect that and do not try to force them.

Perceived vs True Low Milk Supply

Okay, so what if your baby is fussing while latched on or what if they want to latch all the time? It's understandable that, especially since you can't measure exactly how much your baby is taking in, you may have doubts about whether you're making enough.

Remember a few sections ago when we talked about how you can tell that your baby is getting enough milk? That's a huge factor here! If your baby is getting enough milk then that means you're making enough! But what if your baby isn't getting enough milk? Well, that doesn't necessarily mean that you aren't making enough. There are factors that can play into how well your baby removes milk from your chest. So for example, you might produce about 5 ounces per session but maybe your baby is only getting 1 or 2 of those ounces. Don't be alarmed by this! Something as simple as an improper latch can cause your baby to have trouble removing all the milk from your chest, which can easily be fixed by seeing a trained lactation professional. However, other problems like oral ties are a little more complex and require help from a pediatric dentist or ear, nose and throat doctor (ENT). We'll cover more about oral ties in a later section. For now, rest assured that a fussy, cluster feeding or "clingy" baby does not indicate a low milk supply. And just because your baby isn't having enough wet diapers or gaining weight properly doesn't mean your supply is low either!

Pump Output

There is a lot of pressure on new chestfeeding

parents to pump almost around the clock. Unless you are exclusively pumping then there really isn't a need to pump! It's nice to have a small stash in the freezer to use in case of an emergency, or if you leave your baby with a sitter for a few hours, but otherwise there is no need to pump after every feeding like some parents believe they have to. That being said, it can be discouraging, sometimes, if you pump after a feeding and getting as much milk as you thought you would. I wanted to give this topic its own section separate from the one above because of how important it is to remember. Your pump output is *never* a good indication of much milk you are producing. Anywhere from .5 ounces to 4 ounces can be normal for a parent who usually nurses depending on how long it's been since the last time you nursed.

Remember, your body will get used to making milk around the time that your baby usually nurses. If you start pumping only an hour after you've nursed your baby when usually they nurse every 3 hours, don't be alarmed if you get a very small amount of milk. Your body isn't used to producing milk that often!

Another thing to keep in mind is that a pump is a tool created to mimic a baby nursing. So, while it's great for parents who don't want to nurse or need to go back to work, it's artificial and will never be able to remove milk from your chest the way a baby can. This is why you cannot rely on pump output to accurately gauge how much milk you are making. Even though this is a section on its own, it falls right in line with the section above. A low pump output does not mean that you have a low milk supply, especially if your baby has enough diapers and is gaining weight properly!

Power Pumping

Now, let me remind you we will go much further into what oral ties are in a later section. For now, I need to mention that over time oral ties that go undiagnosed and don't get corrected can cause low milk supply. Power pumping is a fantastic way to increase your supply. It won't happen overnight, but give it a few weeks and you should start to see a difference. Here's how you power pump!

Using a double pump (pumping both sides at the same time) Pump for 20 minutes then rest for 10. Pump for 10 minutes then rest for 10 again. Pump for another 10 minutes and you're done! Repeat this 2-3 times a day until you start to see an increase in your baby's wet diapers and weight gain.

What Do I Do with My Pumped Milk?

Whether you're exclusively pumping or just pumping to have a night away from your baby, it's important to know the proper way to store your milk so it doesn't spoil. The best way to keep your milk fresh the longest is by freezing it.

Before freezing your milk make sure that it is in a "food safe" storage container like a bottle, human milk storage bags or silicone molds often used to make ice cubes. I recommend storing them in quantities no larger than 4 ounces, this is the average bottle size for most babies. Freezing too much at one time can cause the unused milk to go bad quicker!

Using a silicone mold is my favorite eco-friendly way to freeze milk because after the cubes are frozen you can place them in a glass jar in the freezer and you don't have to worry about throwing away plastic milk storage bags or having the bottles you need to feed your baby be unavailable. However, choose the method that works best for your family. Frozen milk is good to stay in your normal freeze for 6 months or 12 months in a stand-alone deep freezer so make sure you label your containers!

When you're ready to thaw your milk there are two ways you can do it safely. The first is by putting it in the refrigerator and letting it thaw over the course of a day. If you need the milk faster you can heat up a cup, bowl or pot of warm water. Place the food safe container with the milk still in it, into the container of water. Swirl the container of milk around for about a minute and the milk should start to thaw! Remember, never heat up your milk in the microwave. The microwave can cause hot "pockets" where the milk feels "just right" when you test it but inside the bottle there might be a pocket of milk that is hot enough to burn the baby. If you're not ready to freeze your milk you can leave it in your refrigerator for up to 5 days before it goes bad. Don't panic if you accidentally leave milk on the counter, as long as you put it in the fridge within 4 hours it's still safe for your baby!

A lot of parents also wonder if they are able to mix milk from different pumping sessions. You absolutely can! Just make sure all of the milk is the same temperature so there's no room for bacteria to grow. You can either warm them up separate before mixing, or if you get both of them from the fridge then you can mix them straight from there. As long as you have stored and thawed it properly you can feed your baby milk that is warm or cold!

There's Blood in My Milk!

It's not uncommon to notice milk that is a little pink-ish in color which usually means there's a bit of blood in it. Most of the time it's from a small abrasion on your nipple that you may have not even noticed.

Don't worry, this milk is still perfectly safe for your baby to drink. Think about it this way, if they were nursing straight from your chest, you may not have even noticed it!

Different Colored Milk

Human milk can come in all different colors and luckily most of them are not problematic! Here are all the different colors you may see human milk in and what it means.

Pink- Blood in milk, parent ate beets.
Green- parent ate spinach, seaweed or an herbal vitamin.
Orange- parent ate carrots.
Black- parent is taking antibiotics.
Red/Brown- parent is taking pyridium (medication frequently prescribed for a Urinary Tract Infection (UTI).

If you notice your milk in any of these colors it is still safe for your baby to drink! However, if you notice <u>bright/hot pink milk</u> this can be due to something called *Serratia Marsescens* and is important that you do not feed this to your baby and mention it to your doctor right away as this can be potentially life threatening.

Nutrition for Parents

I often get questions on the type of diet that should be followed when a parent is using their milk to feed their baby. You'll be surprised to learn that there aren't as many restrictions as you might have originally thought.

How Much and What Should I Eat?

Generally speaking, chestfeeding burns about 500 additional calories so, in order to at least maintain your weight and keep up with your new energy needs, consuming about 500 additional calories is recommended. Don't worry if you have trouble increasing your intake though, your body will still make enough of the nutritious milk that your baby needs since your caloric intake doesn't actually change the caloric value of your milk! It's also important to note that caloric intake does not have any bearing on your milk supply either. You will still make plenty of milk even if you don't consume an extra 500 calories. There are parents in 3rd world countries who are malnourished and still produce what their baby needs and, in fact, this is often the only source of nutrition available for their babies. When you're thinking about what to put in your body try to eat foods that are high in vitamins A, B1, B2,B3, B6, B12, C and D as well as fatty acids, zinc and iodine. These are things found in your milk and are important for your baby's development.

Is There Anything I Can't Eat?

I think you'll love the answer to this one. For the

most part there's nothing you can't eat! There's a misconception that foods high in sugar like beans and legumes or high in Sulphur like broccoli that make you gassy will cause your baby to be gassy to. The reality is, these are not things passed through your milk. So eat all the beans, broccoli and legumes you want! Babies, especially newborns, are naturally very gassy because their digestive system is still immature but nothing you eat will have any bearing on that!

Now, there are some circumstances where a baby might have something like a milk protein allergy or soy intolerance in which case you should avoid dairy and soy products, but this is something that needs to be tested by your baby's pediatrician. Sometimes, babies grow out of this so you may not be on this diet forever!

What About Alcohol?

Of course, when we talk about things you can't consume one of the big questions is how much alcohol, if any, can a chestfeeding parent drink? As a general rule of thumb, if you can legally drive a vehicle then it is safe for you to nurse. Alcohol passes through human milk the same way that it passes through blood so pumping and then dumping the milk will not make it pass any quicker. Time is the only thing that will remove the alcohol from your milk and it typically takes about 2-3 hours for every drink. But remember, if you can legally drive then it is safe to nurse!

What Medications Can I take?

You should always make sure you mention to your doctor that you are chestfeeding when they prescribe a new medication so they can prescribe something safe. If you ever have doubts you can check the website "Lactmed" by searching the name of the medication followed by "Lactmed" and clicking the first link. This website provides detailed case studies and information on how medications will pass through your milk and any possible side effects your baby might have.

Things To Look Out For

When I was preparing to nurse my daughter, nothing I read prepared me for the reality that became ours. There were so many warning signs for problems I completely ignored because I had no idea they were even there. When I thought about the type of information I wanted to include in this book, it became very important to me to make sure there was a section on red flags to watch out for, as well as, the not-so-fun parts about chestfeeding.

Oral Ties

As a Certified Breastfeeding Specialist with her own business, the most common problem parents (unknowingly) come to me for is an oral tie. The two types of oral ties that have the greatest impact on a chestfeeding infant are Tongue Ties and Lip Ties. Both can be characterized by a thick, shiny and/or inelastic oral frenulum either under the upper lip or under the tongue. While tongue ties are more problematic, lip ties are usually what get noticed first by a parent. It's important to note that because of the way the jaw and skull form while your baby is in utero, when there is a lip tie present there is almost always a tongue tie, as well.

So what's the big deal with oral ties? Why do they cause so many problems? Well, Lip Ties restrict your baby's ability to flange their top tip out properly, making it difficult to get a proper seal on your chest when they are latched on. Tongue Ties restrict the tongue's range of mobility, making it difficult for your baby to move their tongue in a way that supports the efficient removal of milk from your chest. This means that over-time, your milk supply may start to decrease because even though you might be producing 5 ounces a session, your baby can only remove 2 of those ounces so then your body starts making 2 ounces a session but your baby can only remove .5 ounces and so on.

Now, what are the signs of an oral tie? What should you be looking out for? Some of the most obvious signs are dehydration, slow or no weight gain and a low diaper count, but others include "colic" (inconsolable crying), clicking sound while nursing, unusual sleep patterns, excess spit-up, excess gas and in older children speech impediments and delays. Before we knew what we know now about oral ties, the solution used to be to just give the baby a bottle and the parent would be told that chestfeeding was impossible for them. However, even if that were true, there are still long term effects of living with an oral tie. As a toddler they can cause frequent gagging and choking on solid food, speech delays and a gap in the front teeth. Well into adulthood, they can cause speech impediments, chronic muscle stiffness and pain in your shoulders, neck and jaw and even chronic migraines. I always tell the parents I work with to get the oral ties corrected even if they don't continue to chestfeed because preventing some of these long term effects is well worth it.

Unfortunately, as you may have gathered from reading part one of this book, most pediatricians have no idea what an oral tie is or how to identify them. The same is true about pediatric dentists and ENTs. They aren't always trained to identify all four classes of ties or correct them properly. So, how do you get your child assessed for oral ties? Well, you can start by looking for an IBCLC or CBS in your area. If you are a Women, Infant and Children (WIC) participant, they offer these services for free! You can also join your area's local Tongue Tie Support Group on Facebook and post that you're looking for a provider. These groups are ran by IBCLCs and sometimes even the providers themselves, so you can look at reviews from other parents and decide which one is best for you based on insurance compatibility and location!

The procedure to get an oral tie corrected is a very quick one! No exaggeration here, it takes an average of 1 minute and 30 sections. Your provider may either use scissors or a laser to release the tie and then they will direct you on how to do the aftercare which usually involves doing tongue and/or lip stretches. In more severe instances where an oral tie didn't get corrected until the child was much older speech and/or physical therapy may be required.

It's important to know the warning signs of an oral tie so you can get it corrected as soon as possible. Doing so will not only save your chestfeeding relationship, but help to prevent any of these long term side effects!

Fast/Powerful Letdown

Sometimes, parents have a fast or powerful letdown which basically means instead of a slow trickle or gentle stream of milk coming out, it can feel more like a waterfall to a baby. This may sometimes cause your baby to have an aversion to your chest because it may be too much for them to handle. Now this doesn't mean that you can't chestfeed anymore! There are luckily some tricks you can try to make a letdown like this easier on your baby.

Some parents have luck with pumping for a few minutes before latching their baby. Doing this means there won't be as sudden of a letdown when your baby latches because you will have pumped through most of the letdown. Pumping before every nursing session can get tiresome and overwhelming, so I always recommend the alternative of trying new nursing positions! Two positions that can help soften a letdown are nursing on your side and nursing while laying back. Both positions use gravity as an advantage, making it harder for the milk to flow downward faster!

Luckily, the older your baby gets, the more they may be able to tolerate a letdown like this. You may not have to worry about it for your entire chestfeeding journey!

Foremilk/Hindmilk

It's a very common misconception that human milk is made up of two components, "foremilk" and "hindmilk." These are simply the terms to describe milk at the beginning of a nursing or pumping session and milk at the end of a nursing or pumping session.

Typically, the milk at the beginning of a session is higher in water and lactose, whereas the milk at the end of a session is higher in fat. However, there is no "magic moment" where your milk changes from foremilk to hindmilk. All of the milk you produce is created just for your baby and is perfect for them!

Milk Blebs

Milk Blebs are blocked nipple pores (different from milk ducts) and often appear on the nipple as something that looks like an ingrown hair. They are fairly common and usually easy to treat. If caught early, you can use home remedies like salt water soaks and gentle massages to break up the blockage. On rare occasions you may need to have it drained by a healthcare professional.

Clogged Milk Ducts

Clogged milk ducts are something that can happen fairly frequently and is a result of milk not being properly extracted from your chest. If your baby isn't latched properly or if they have orals, this can be the cause of them not extracting milk properly.

When this happens, you may experience swelling and redness as well as pain during and between nursing/pumping sessions.

Luckily, the remedy to this problem is pretty simple! You want to get that trapped milk out so latch and pump as frequently as possible. Using a warm compress or hot water in the shower can help break up that milk and make it easier to let it escape. You can also use a Haakaa filled with warm salt water to help bring that milk down and soothe the pain.

Watch for a fever and flu like symptoms, clogged ducts have the potential to turn into mastitis. If you experience a fever and flu like symptoms, call your healthcare provider as soon as possible.

Mastitis

This infection, most common in the upper outer quadrant of the chest, occurs in up to 20% of lactating people in the first 6 months. It is, typically, the result of prolonged engorgement and/or extreme stress on the chest, such as wearing clothing, a binder or bra that is too tight or for too long. You may experience a fever and flu-like symptoms as well as a painful, lump and hard chest. If you are pumping, you may also notice your milk may look lumpy or gelatin-like and also contain blood.

It is important to empty the chest fully and often when mastitis is diagnosed, and though your milk may look different it is still completely safe for your littleone to drink. It should be noted, however, that milk from the infected side may taste a little salty as milk with mastitis has about twice the amount of sodium. If your baby does not like the taste, pump you milk as often as your baby would nurse and save it for milk baths!

Mastitis should be treated with a full course of antibiotics if the symptoms persist after 24 hours.

Please make sure you are in constant contact with your healthcare provider, so that they can monitor you and decide if antibiotics are necessary.

Aside from antibiotics, a parent who is fighting mastitis should always try to rest as much as possible, keep a warm compress on whenever they can, drink plenty of water and drain the chest often.

Thrush

Thrush is a fungal infection that is often passed back and forth from baby to parent through nursing. You may experience sharp, hot, stabbing-like pain in your nipple and/or chest and may notice white patches in your baby's mouth, especially on their tongue.

Thankfully, as long as the pain is not too unbearable and you baby still wants to nurse, it is completely safe to continue nursing while being treated for thrush. Just be sure to have you doctor treat both you and your baby at the same time, otherwise you will continue to pass it back and forth.

Postpartum Depression & Psychosis

Rarely talked about, but often experienced, postpartum depression occurs in about 10-20% of birthing people. This is characterized by -- feelings of intense sadness, guilt, irritability, rage, difficulty with baby, lack of motivation, and insomnia or extreme fatigue. In extreme cases, such as with postpartum psychosis, a parent may even have thoughts of harming themselves or their baby, hallucinations, and erratic outbursts of violent behavior. This is something many parents are afraid to admit they are experiencing.

It's so important to remember these thoughts and feelings are not you and are the result of the rapid rise and fall of hormones after you give birth. If at any point in time you feel like you might be experiencing postpartum depression, please let your doctor know. A combination of therapy and medication, as well as, a little extra support from family and friends can do wonders and really help to bring you out from under that cloud.

Dysphoric Milk Ejection Reflex

Often misdiagnosed as postpartum depression, dysphoric milk ejection reflex (DMER) is characterized by feelings of hopelessness, sadness, anger and distress, intrusive thoughts or thoughts of self-harm, and/or intense paranoia only during the milk ejection reflex, or let-down. It does not last for the entire nursing session and these things are not experienced before or after nursing.

Research on this condition is limited because it is a fairly new discovery. At the moment, there is no known treatment for it, but some studies suggest that foods high in tyrosine and phenylalanine (such as certain beans and legumes) may help. Since new information is constantly being released, it's always a good idea to check with your doctor about what treatments may become available for you.

Final Thoughts

Chest-feeding, though natural, is not always easy. It's not uncommon for parents to experience obstacles, whether it is their first or fourth time around. I hope after having read through all of this information, you feel more prepared for any obstacles that may come your way. I hope you found comfort in reading stories from people just like you, knowing that you are not alone in whatever you went through or are still going through. I'm honored to have had you as my reader, to have told my story and others like it... and most importantly, to have held space for you.

Resources Mentioned

For more information on the Baby Friendly Initiative and how to find a baby friendly hospital near you, you can visit their website: *https://www.babyfriendlyusa.org/about/*

If you would like to have a look at the two growth charts that pediatricians may use to measure your little one, you can find that information the CDC's website: *https://www.cdc.gov/growthcharts/who_charts.htm*

Glossary

Here you will find a list of definitions for terms found throughout this book. This glossary is organized in alphabetical order starting with "B".

B

Bili Lights

A type of light therapy (phototherapy) used to treat newborn jaundice (a yellow coloring of the skin and eyes caused by abnormal bilirubin levels).

Bilirubin

An orange-yellow pigment formed in the liver.

Binder

An article of clothing worn on the upper chest by people who wish to make their chest appear flatter.

BIPOC

An acronym for "Black, Indiginous, People of Color," used to describe the population that does not fall under the race of "White".

Breast Shells

Hollow, lightweight plastic disks worn inside the shirt to help correct flat or inverted nipples.

C

CBS
An acronym for Certified Breastfeeding Specialist.

Colicky
A word used to describe an infant that cries inconsolably for seemingly no reason.

Colostrum
The first form of human milk that is produced after delivery. It is thick and yellow in color compared to mature milk which is thinner and white/off-white in color.

E

ENT
An acronym for Ear Nose and Throat Specialist/Doctor

F

Fenugreek
A type of herb native to the Mediterranean, southern Europe and west Asian. It is commonly used in Indian cuisine as well as herbal medicine around the world.

H

Haakaa
A hands-free, silicone milk pump that uses suction to pull milk from the chest.

Heteronormative
The idea that heterosexuality is the default and preferred expression of sexual orientation.

I

IBCLC
An acronym for international board certified lactation consultant.

ICAN
An acronym for International Cesarean Awareness Network

IUI
An acronym for intrauterine insemination -- a procedure where sperm is placed directly into the uterus while a person is ovulating.

IVF
An acronym for in-vitro fertilization -- a process where egg and sperm are combined outside the body to create an embryo which is then placed inside of a uterus.

L

Latinx
An inclusive way to describe someone and a group of people from Latin American descent.

N

NICU
An acronym for Neonatal Intensive Care Unit -- a unit in most hospitals where newborn babies who need intensive care are taken to.

Nipple Graft
The reconstruction of a person's areola and nipples using skin from other parts of the body (usually the chest) after

Nipple Shield
A lightweight, plastic disk that can be placed on the nipple to make it easier for babies to latch on. Oftentimes these are used for premature babies with smaller mouths, babies with oral ties or for babies whose parent has flat or inverted nipples.

Non-Binary
A term used by someone who does not feel that they fit into either of the binary gender expressions of "male" or "female".

O

Orofacial Myologist
a professional with a speech-language pathology, dental or dental hygiene clinical background.

P

Pitocin
A hormone that causes the uterus to contract, used when inducing labor in pregnant people.

Polyamorous
A term used to describe;

1. a person who participates in multiple romantic relationships, with the consent of all parties involved
2. a romantic relationship that includes multiple people.

Polycystic Ovarian Syndrome (PCOS)
A condition where a person's ovaries produce an abnormal amount of male sex hormones when they are typically found in small amount in people assigned female at birth.

Posterior Tongue Tie
A type of oral tie (tongue tie) that is furthest back in the mouth. Sometimes also classified as a "type 4" tongue tie.

R

REF (reflexe d'ejection fort) (Overactive let down)
An acronym for Reflexe D'Ejection Fort, French for "strong ejection reflex" a term used to describe when a lactating parent has an overactive, fast and/or powerful milk letdown when pumping or nursing. In English we call this an "Overactive" letdown.

S

SNS
An acronym for Supplemental Nursing System -- a device used to help a parent supplement their baby's nutrient intake with additional human milk or formula while they are nursing at the chest.

T

Top Surgery
A surgery that is performed on the chest as part of gender reassignment where breast tissue is removed to give a more masculine appearance of the chest.

Trans
An umbrella term used to describe someone who does not identify as the same gender they were assigned at birth.

W

WIC
An acronym for Women, Infants and Children -- a program in the United States that works to provide food and lactation support for low income families.

Made in the USA
Las Vegas, NV
23 January 2023

66134444R00085